Surgicalillustration.com

Suturing Part 1:

The Principles and Techniques of Tying Surgical Knots

I0032187

D. OUDIT

Consultant Plastic and Reconstructive Surgeon
Christie Hospital, Manchester UK

M. BRIGGS

Senior Medical Artist
President of the Medical Artists Association of Great Britain

Suturing Part 1:
The Principles and Techniques of Tying Surgical Knots

Copyright © 2015 by Surgicalillustration.com

ISBN 978-0-9574996-1-4

Dedications

This book is dedicated to my loving and supporting wife, Michelle, who gives me the strength I need to face the many challenges of life.

DO

This book is dedicated to Vicky and Lucas and I thank them for their support throughout this project.

MB

Table of Contents

Surgicalillustration.com

SUTURING Part 1: The Principles and Techniques of Tying Knots
D. Oudit | M. Briggs

Preface

The techniques of tying knots and suturing are an art that every doctor and surgical practitioner should master. Before one embarks on suturing, one should be confident in tying stable surgical knots. This is best done on simulated models before actually performing it on patients. Fortunately, with the advance in medical education, there is much deserved emphasis currently being placed in skill stations. A book of this type, which outlines the most basic skills of surgical practice, is a good companion to students, trainees and residents to complement their practical sessions.

We all, to some extent, learn various things differently. For some, tying knots and suturing comes naturally without a concerted effort to study the subject. And for others, trying to learn the techniques of hand-tying a knot is a whole lot more difficult. This book was designed in a very illustrative manner so that it could be easily skimmed through or could be studied in a bit of detail before attempting the practical exercises in a simulated environment.

This series is divided into two volumes. In this volume, we hope that the reader would learn and master the techniques of tying stable while at the same time being able to recognize unstable knots and the techniques that creates these. In this way, the reader can aim to always create stable knots and avoid unstable ones.

SurgicalIllustration.com

SUTURING Part 1: The Principles and Techniques of Tying Knots
D. Oudit | M. Briggs

In the second volume, we aim to teach the reader techniques of suturing and applications for the various types.

We sincerely hope that this book would be adequate to help students and health care practitioners to learn and master the art of tying knots.

DO & MB

Manchester , UK

2015.

Prologue

This is the first of a two-part series on suturing. It outlines the techniques of tying knots by employing visual photographs of the steps of the procedures to complement the text. Illustrations are also included where the authors believe that these would aid in the description of the technique or to explain the result.

Each chapter begins with an, 'Introduction' that seeks to highlight the important characteristics of the particular type of knot. This is then followed by a series of pictorial step-by-step instructions helping the reader to visually appreciate the techniques.

In the description of each type of knot, a simulated suture material (a string with a red and a white end) is used. To standardize the description, the red end of the suture is held by the left hand and the white end by the right hand. This is particularly applicable to left-handed readers. Readers who are right-handed may wish to reverse the order of the suture ends and work with the red end held by the right hand and the white end by the left hand. In such cases, the instructions should be interpreted appropriately.

SurgicalIllustration.com

SUTURING Part 1: The Principles and Techniques of Tying Knots
D. Oudit | M. Briggs

Photos and illustrations are included to highlight the configurations of the knots at the end of the appropriate chapters.

Acknowledgements

We are extremely grateful for the loving support of families during the preparation of the manuscript for this work. We are also infinitely indebted to our many teachers in the past whose skills and dedicated have been the basis of this work.

Surgicalillustration.com

SUTURING Part 1: The Principles and Techniques of Tying Knots
D. Oudit | M. Briggs

CHAPTER 1
INTRODUCTION

Suturing is a basic technique operative technique in surgery which every medical student and doctor should master. In order to master the technique, one needs to learn the skills of knot tying. A wound repaired by suturing is only as strong as the suture material and skill of the surgeon who performed it. One of the most important skills to be mastered in this regard is the creation of stable knots.

This book takes the reader through various techniques for tying knots (both hand-tying and instrument-tying, as appropriate). The stable knots are distinguished from the unstable knots.

For a beginner, learning these skills can pose as a daunting challenge. It is not easily taught either. So therefore, this book aims to teach the reader these techniques using as much visual aid as possible. It is the intention that the reader will study the contents of this book while practising the techniques at the same time. This is then likely to produce the optimal benefit for the reader.

SurgicalIllustration.com

SUTURING Part 1: The Principles and Techniques of Tying Knots
D. Oudit | M. Briggs

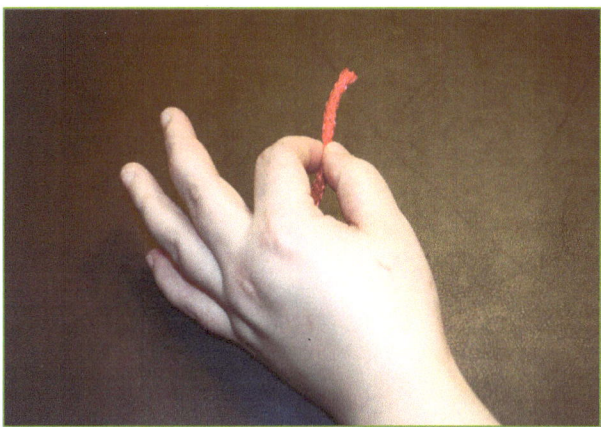

Figure 1.1: Pronation of the left hand.

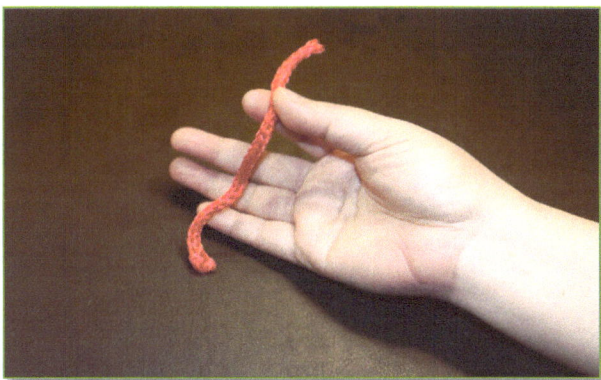

Figure 1.2: Supination of the right hand.

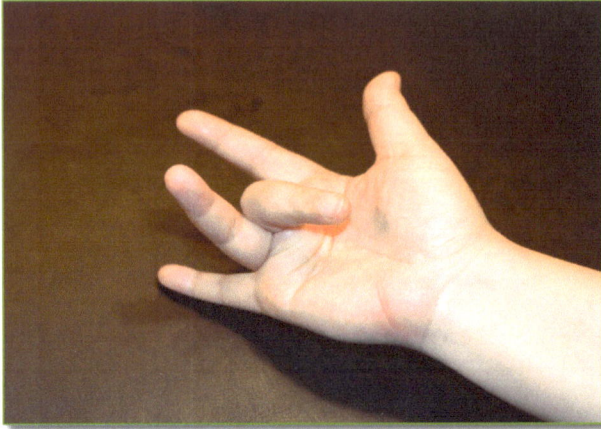

Figure 1.3: Flexion of the right middle finger.

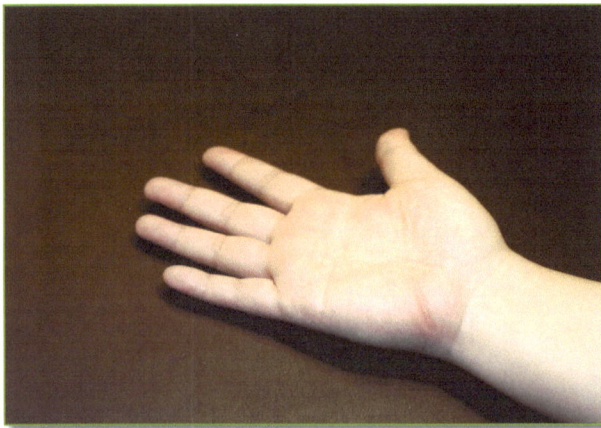

Figure 1.4: Extension of the fingers of the right hand.

CHAPTER 2
CLASSIFICATION OF KNOTS

A knot is defined as a fastening made by looping a length of suture material on itself and tightening it.

Although in the current context it is mostly applied to surgical knots, the art of tying knots has been advanced by members of other professions bearing little or no commonality with surgery, such as fishermen.

Knots maybe formed by a hand-tying technique or maybe instrument tied.

SurgicalIllustration.com

SUTURING Part 1: The Principles and Techniques of Tying Knots
D. Oudit | M. Briggs

Knots maybe classified based on the location in relation to the surface of the skin, on the technique used in its creation or on the degree of its stability. The degree of stability of a knot is directly dependent on the technique used in its formation.

- ### *Anatomical location*

In its most simple form, surgical knots may be classified as external or buried knots. External knots are formed and lie above the level of the surface of the skin even though the actually suture material penetrates the skin. Buried knots are formed and lie below the surface of the skin.

- ### *Technique employed in tying knot*

There are various techniques that are used in the formation of knots. The knots formed are different in physical configuration for each technique used. Some of the commonly used knots are listed below:

- Simple knot
- Square knot
- Surgeon's knot
- Granny knot

14

- *Knot Stability*

In general, knots are deemed as either stable or unstable. Most knots however, would display a certain degree of stability. Examples of stable knots are the square knot and the surgeon's knot. Examples of unstable knots are the simple knot and the granny knots. Unstable knots are undesirable in surgical practice and therefore not recommended.

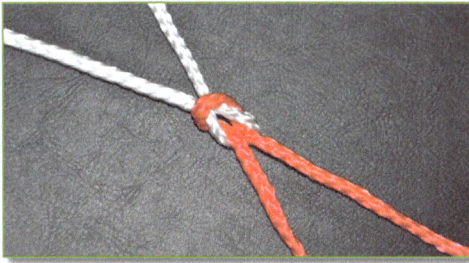

Figure 2.1: A configuration of a stable knot

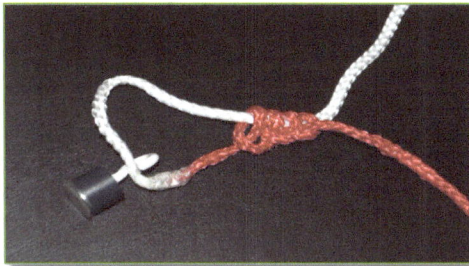

Figure 2.2: A configuration of an unstable knot

CHAPTER 3

PROPERTIES OF THE IDEAL KNOT

The properties of a knot are important when considering the potential effects of the knot/suture material on the tissues of the body.

Knots are formed from suture materials that are foreign to the tissues of the body. These therefore, invoke an inflammatory response that affects the overall outcome of the resultant scar.

Also, knots need to be as stable as possible so that they do not unravel at the critical stages of wound healing since this may lead to wound dehiscence.

The ideal knot should therefore invoke the least inflammatory response possible.

In order to achieve this, it should have the following characteristics:

1. **Knot Volume:** The knot should be least bulky as possible especially buried knots as these make maximal contact with the tissues. This reduces the inflammatory reaction of the tissues to the suture material.

2. **Tension:** Excessive tension on the suture material should be avoided as much as possible as this may strangulate the tissue resulting in tissue ischaemia, infarction, necrosis and infection.

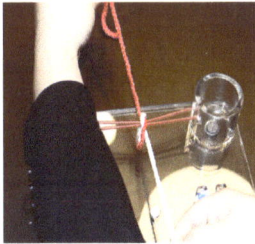

Figure 3.1: Less bulky first throw of simple square knot

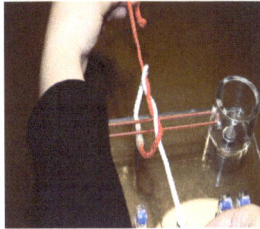

Figure 3.2: More bulky fist throw of a 'surgeon's' knot.

SurgicalIllustration.com

SUTURING Part 1: The Principles and Techniques of Tying Knots
D. Oudit | M. Briggs

The ideal knot should be as stable as possible and the minimal length of suture material should be used to achieve this maximal stability. In order to achieve this, the knot should have the following characteristics:

1. **Knot Configuration:** The configuration of the knot should lend to its inherent stability to avoid knot slippage. The knot should be laid down firmly to avoid unloosening.

2. **Knot Size:** The knot should be as compact as possible. The more compact a knot is means that the suture-suture contact is greater. This increases the stability of the knot. Therefore, the ideal knot should be the most stable knot formed that requires the least suture material as possible in its formation.

3. **Technique:** When tying knots, equal tension and counter-tension should be applied to both ends of the suture material in a horizontal plane.

SurgicalIllustration.com

SUTURING Part 1: The Principles and Techniques of Tying Knots
D. Oudit | M. Briggs

4. **Tension:** Excessive tension on the suture material should be avoided as much as possible as this may weaken the suture material leading to breakage. This maybe immediate or delayed, either way, associated with a disastrous outcome.

SurgicalIllustration.com

SUTURING Part 1: The Principles and Techniques of Tying Knots
D. Oudit | M. Briggs

CHAPTER 4

THE SIMPLE KNOT

INTRODUCTION

- ✓ This is an incomplete knot consisting of a single throw.
- ✓ It is therefore unstable.
- ✓ It usually forms the first throw or part of most knots. It is not functional on its own.
- ✓ The ends of the suture material are crossed over each other such that the ends of the suture material end up on opposite sides from where they started off.
- ✓ In order to achieve this, the suture ends are pulled with equal tension in opposite directions in a plane parallel to the horizontal surface of the surface of the skin.

The following figures demonstrate the technique of hand-tying a simple knot step by step.

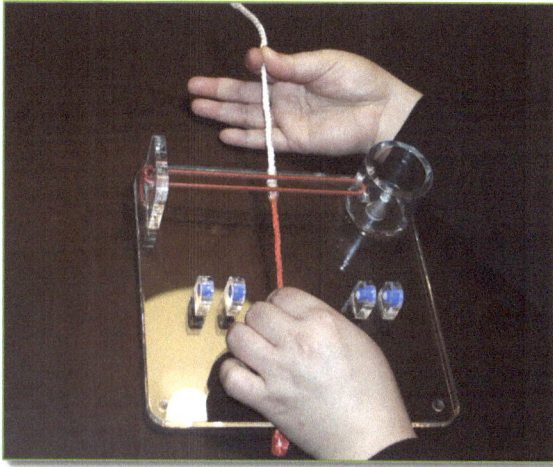

Step 1. The red end of the suture is held firmly between the thumb and index finger of the left hand in the pronated position. The white end of the suture is held firmly between the thumb and index finger of the right hand in the supinated position.

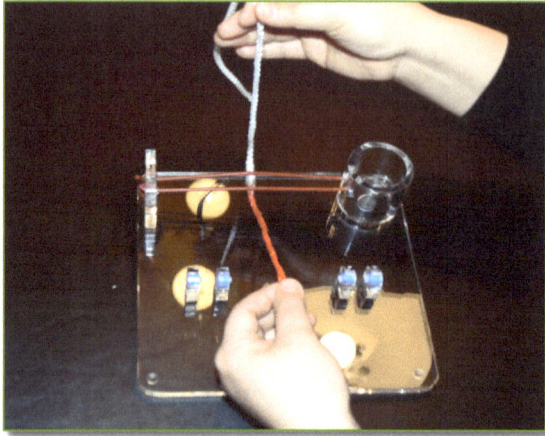

Step 2. Both hands are moved towards the middle of the field.

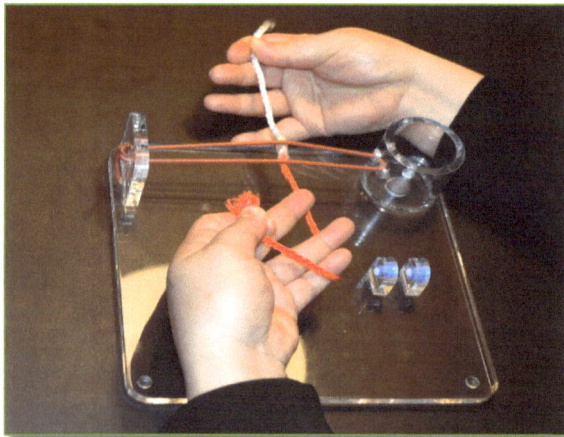

Step 3. The left hand is supinated with the red suture looping around the ulnar side of the little finger.

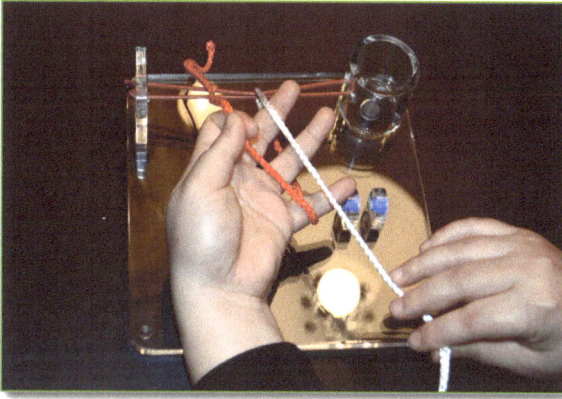

Step 4. The white end is brought to overlie the extended middle, ring and little fingers as shown.

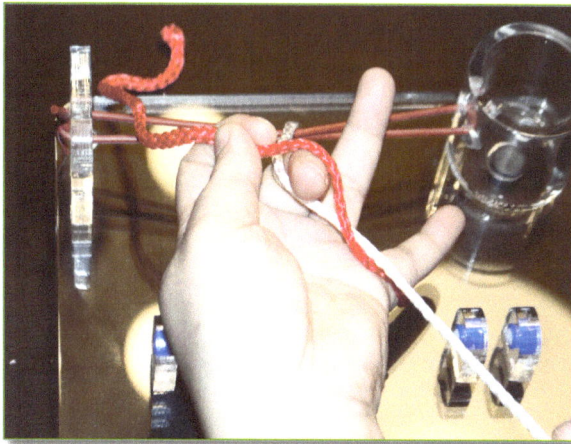

Step 5. The left middle finger is flexed over the white end and under the red end.

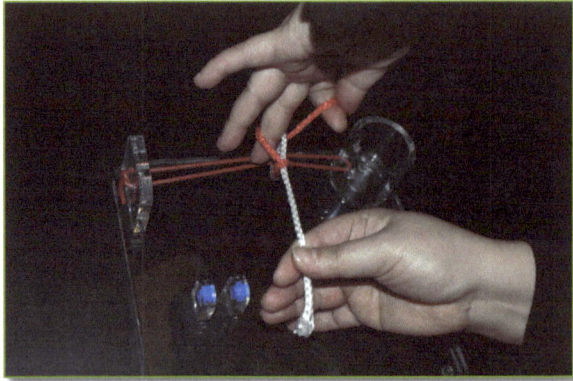

Step 6. The left hand is then pronated.

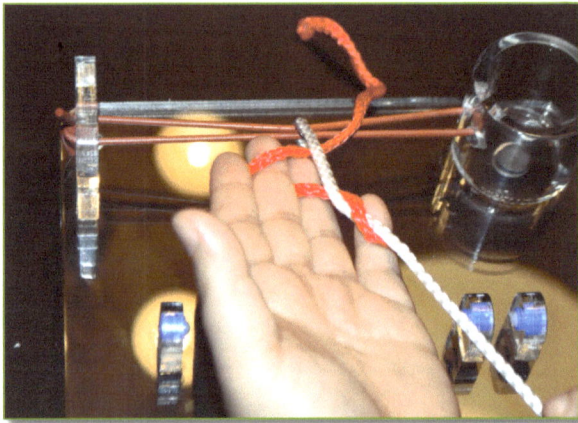

Step 7. The red end is then released by the left thumb and grasp between the left index and middle fingers. The left hand is then pronated and the left middle finger is passed under the white suture to grasp the end of the red suture. The red end is then brought under the white end.

SUTURING Part 1: The Principles and Techniques of Tying Knots
D. Oudit | M. Briggs

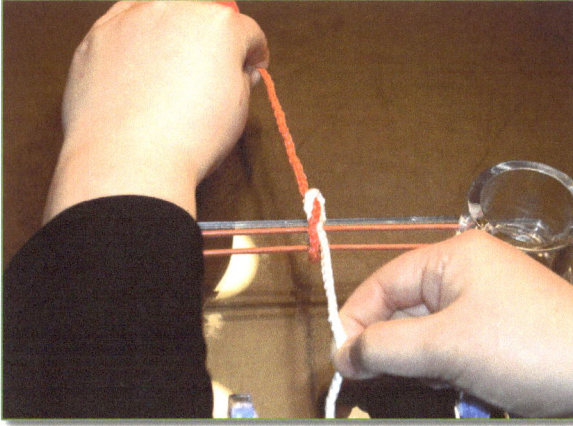

Step 8. Equal horizontal tension is then applied to both ends with the white end being pulled towards the operator and the red end away from the operator. Note that the ends are now on the opposite sides from where they initially started. Also, note that the knot is 'sitting' flat.

The following figures demonstrate the technique of tying a simple knot using a haemostatic clamp or needle-holding forceps in a step-by-step fashion.

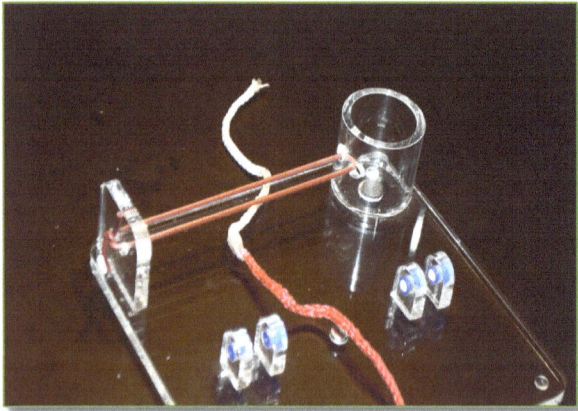

Step 1. The red end of the suture is held by the left hand while the white end of the suture is left free.

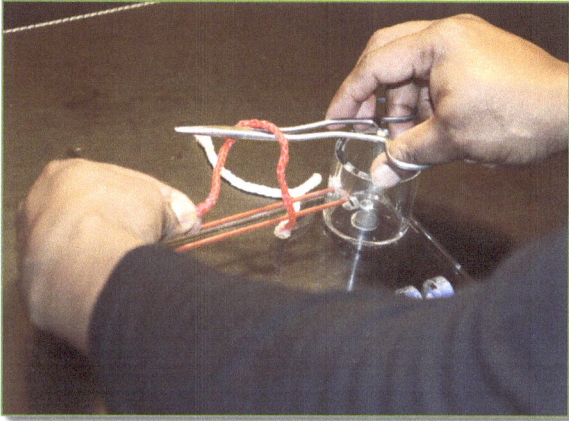

Step 2. The red end is pulled towards the operator making the white end shorter. The red end is looped around the tip of the haemostatic clamp in an anti-clockwise direction.

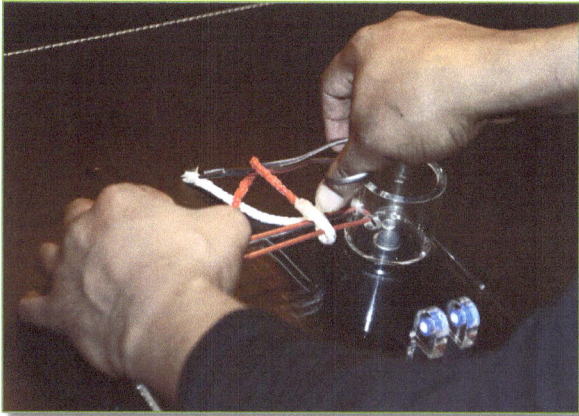

Step 3. The white end is then grasp by the tip of the haemostat.

SurgicalIllustration.com

SUTURING Part 1: The Principles and Techniques of Tying Knots
D. Oudit | M. Briggs

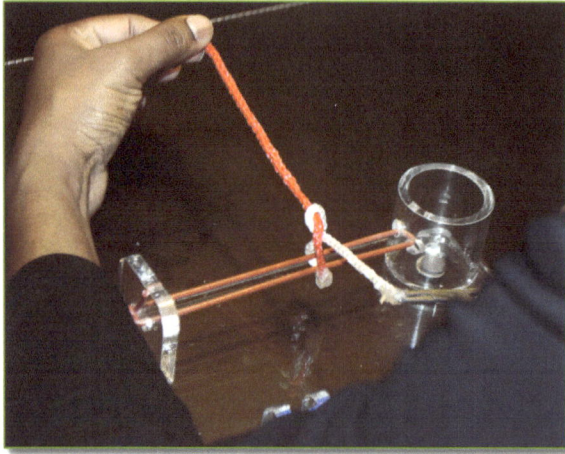

Step 4. Equal and horizontal tension is then applied to both ends with the white end being pulled towards the operator and the red end away from the operator. Note that the ends are now on opposite sides from they initially started.

This is the first throw completed.

This completes the **simple knot** that is incomplete and unstable. Please proceed to next chapter, which describes the square knot that is a complete and stable knot.

CHAPTER 5

THE SQUARE KNOT

- ✓ The square knot is also known as a flat knot or a reef knot.
- ✓ A square knot is a stable and reliable knot.
- ✓ It has symmetry and maximises suture-suture contact per unit area hence resulting in its stability.
- ✓ Stability is achieved with a minimum of two throws. Each throw is similar to a simple knot. However, each throw is done in opposite directions to each other throw.

The following figures demonstrate the technique of hand-tying a square knot step by step. Steps 1 to 8 are the same for the simple knot. *(Please refer to pages 21 - 25)*

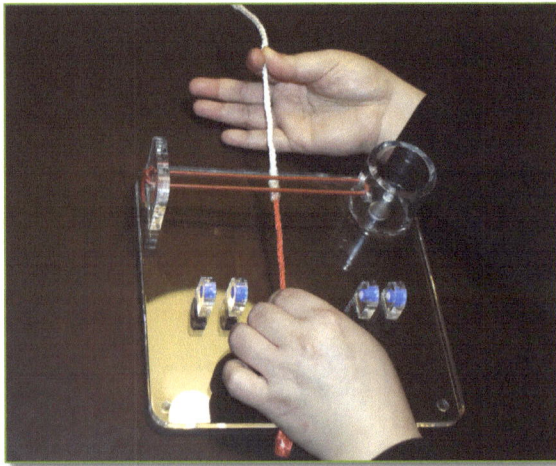

Step 1. The red end of the suture is held firmly between the thumb and index finger of the left hand in the pronated position. The white end of the suture is held firmly between the thumb and index finger of the right hand in the supinated position.

SurgicalIllustration.com

SUTURING Part 1: The Principles and Techniques of Tying Knots
D. Oudit | M. Briggs

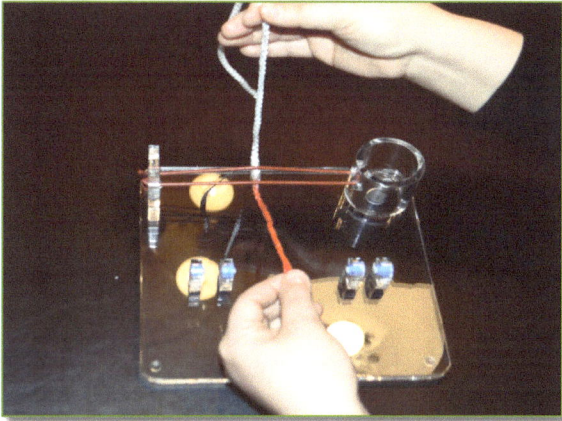

Step 2. Both hands are moved towards the middle of the field.

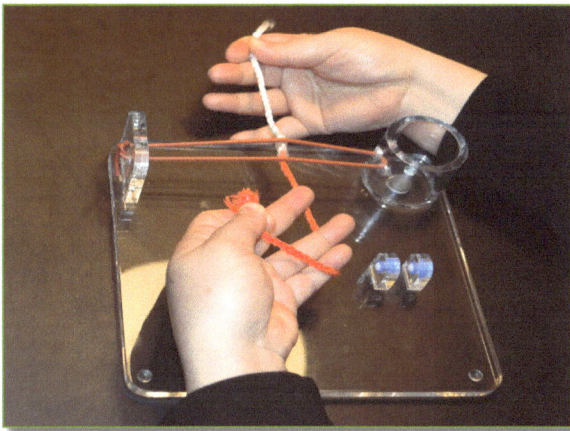

Step 3. The left hand is supinated with the red suture looping around the ulnar side of the little finger.

SurgicalIllustration.com

SUTURING Part 1: The Principles and Techniques of Tying Knots
D. Oudit | M. Briggs

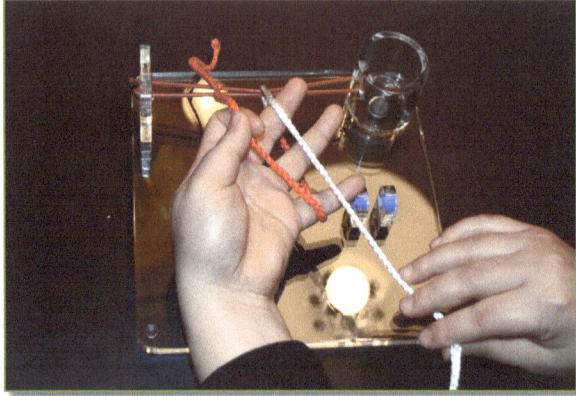

Step 4. The white end is brought to overlie the extended middle, ring and little fingers as shown.

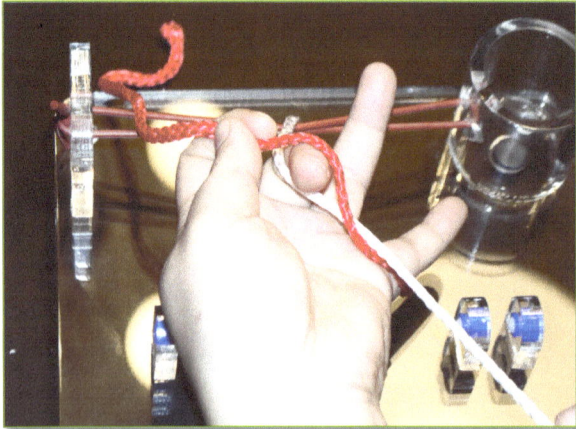

Step 5. The left middle finger is flexed over the white end and under the red end.

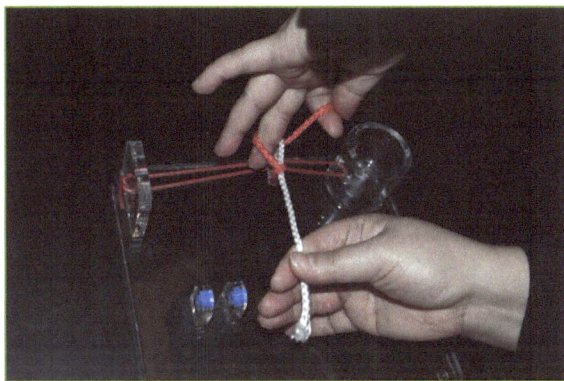

Step 6. The left hand is then pronated.

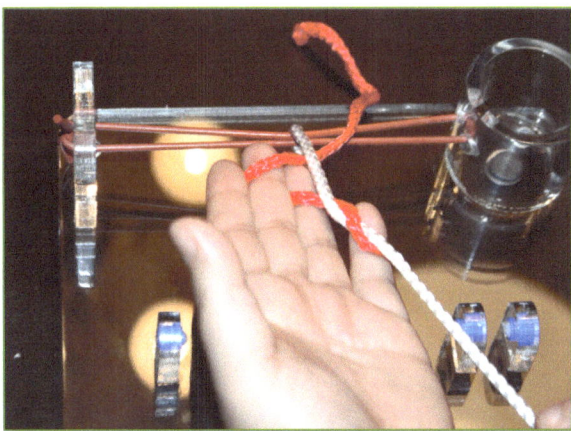

Step 6. The red end is then released by the left thumb and grasp between the left index and middle fingers. The left hand is then pronated and the left middle finger is passed under the white suture to grasp the end of the red suture. The red end is then brought under the white end.

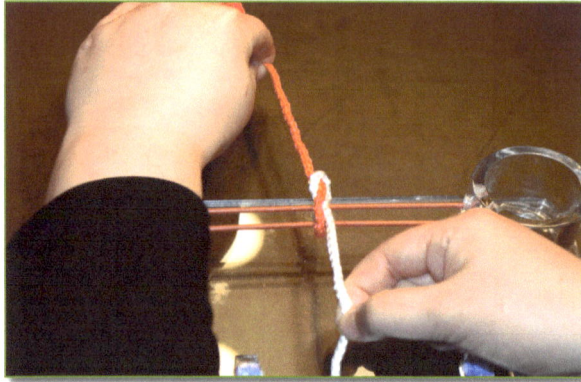

Step 7. Equal horizontal tension is then applied to both ends with the white end being pulled towards the operator and the red end away from the operator.

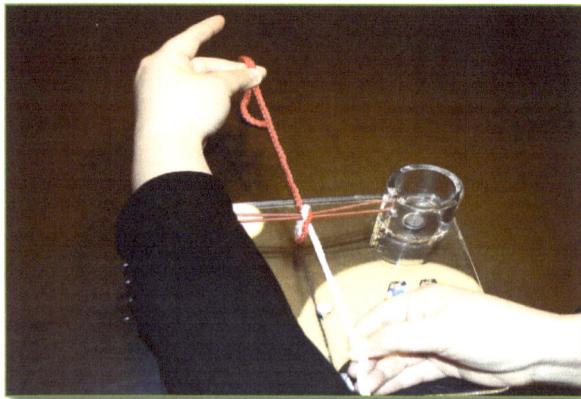

Step 8. The red end is now held between the left thumb and middle finger with the left hand in a pronated position. The white end is held between the right thumb and index finger with the right hand in a pronated position.

SUTURING Part 1: The Principles and Techniques of Tying Knots
D. Oudit | M. Briggs

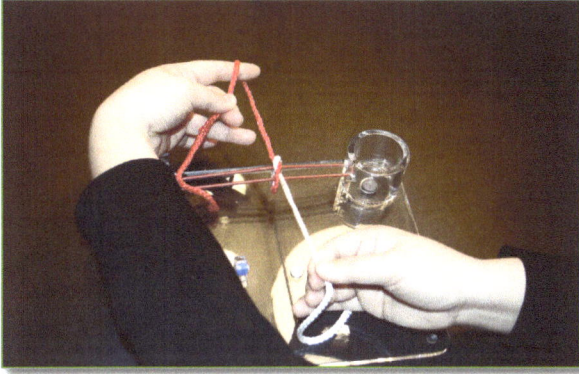

Step 9. The red and is then hooked over the left index finger and brought towards to the middle of the field.

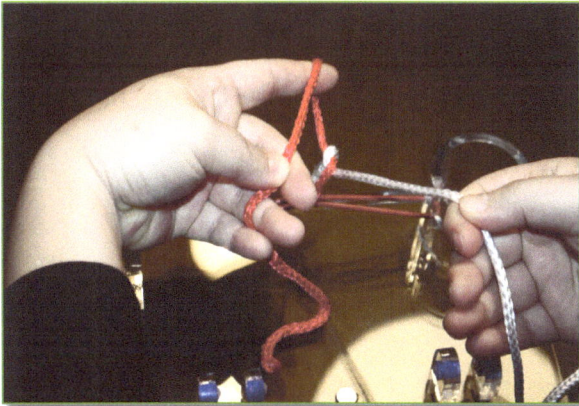

Step 10. The white end is also brought towards the middle of the field.

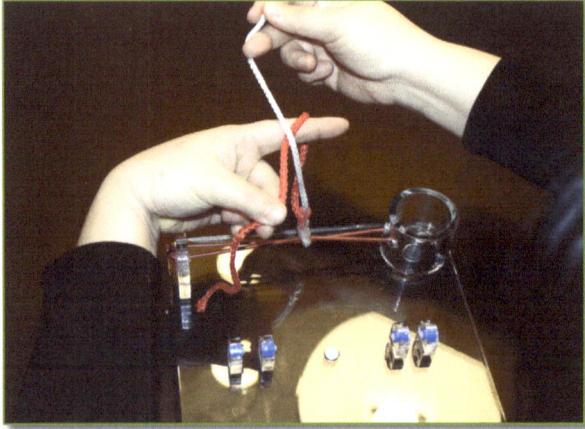

Step 11. The white end is brought to lie over the tip of the left index finger to cross over the red end of the suture material.

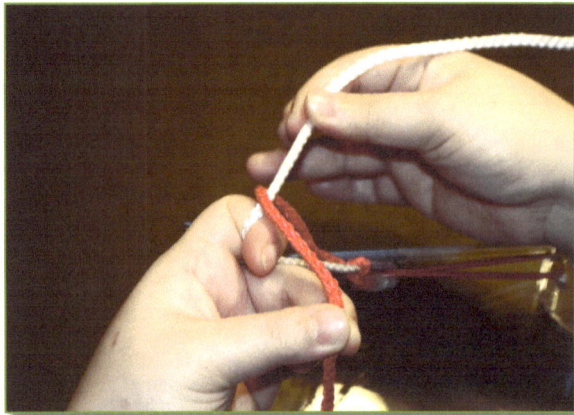

Step 12. The left index finger is then flexed over the white end pulling it inward and then extended over the red end to bring it under the white end.

SurgicalIllustration.com

SUTURING Part 1: The Principles and Techniques of Tying Knots
D. Oudit | M. Briggs

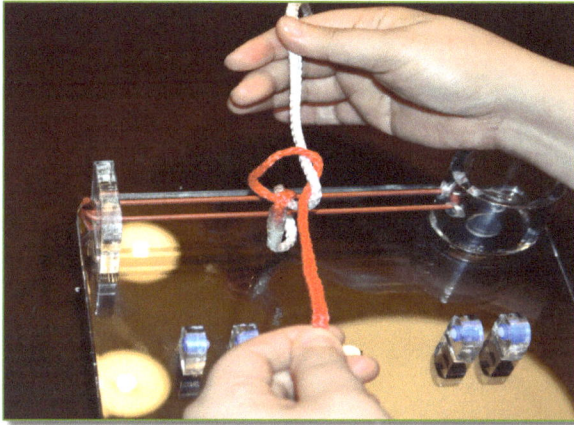

Step 13. The red end is then released from the left thumb and middle fingers and the end pulled through under the white end. Equal and horizontal tension is then applied with the red pulled towards the operator and the white away from the operator.

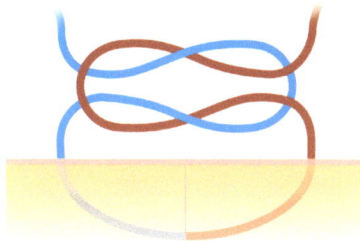

Figure 5.1: An illustration to demonstrate the configuration of the square knot.

SurgicalIllustration.com

SUTURING Part 1: The Principles and Techniques of Tying Knots
D. Oudit | M. Briggs

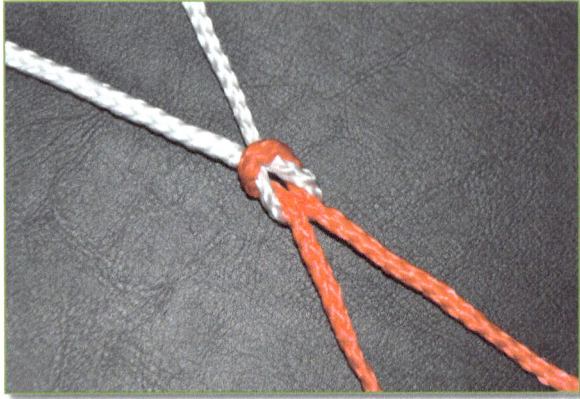

Figure 5.2. Note that the knot has both a symmetric and stable configuration.

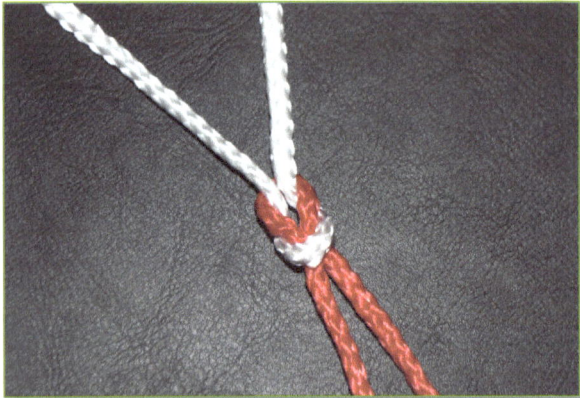

Figure 5.3. Note that the knot has both a symmetric and stable configuration.

The following figures demonstrate the technique of tying a square knot using a haemostatic clamp or needle-holding forceps in a step-by-step fashion.

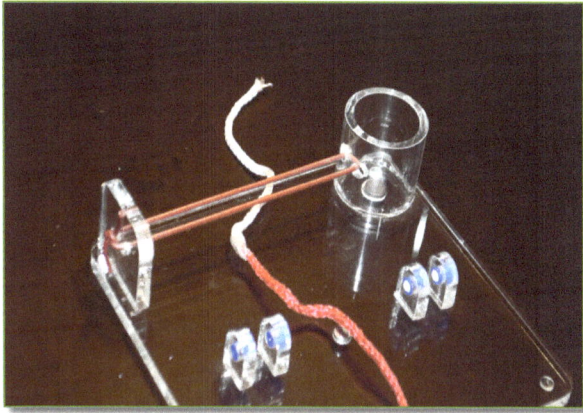

Step 1. The red end of the suture is held by the left hand while the white end of the suture is left free.

SurgicalIllustration.com

SUTURING Part 1: The Principles and Techniques of Tying Knots
D. Oudit | M. Briggs

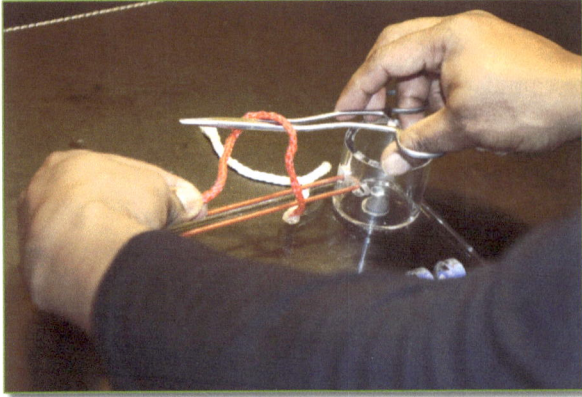

Step 2. The red end is pulled towards the operator making the white end shorter. The red end is looped around the tip of the haemostatic clamp in an anti-clockwise direction.

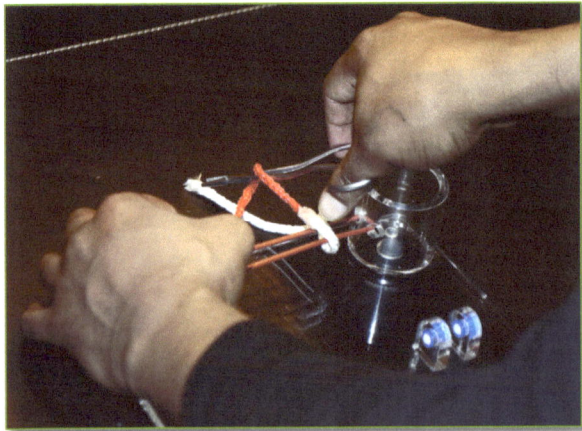

Step 3. The white end is then grasp by the tip of the haemostat.

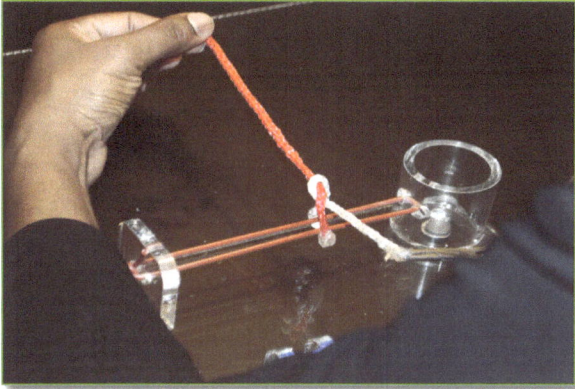

Step 4. Equal and horizontal tension is then applied to both ends with the white end being pulled towards the operator and the red end away from the operator. Note that the ends are now on opposite sides from they initially started.

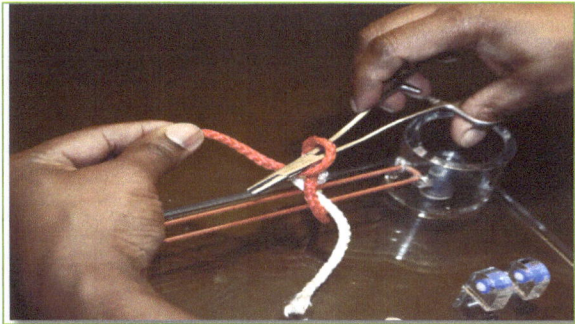

Step 5. The white end of the suture is then released from the tip of the haemostat and the red end is looped around the tip of the haemostatic clamp in a clockwise direction.

SurgicalIllustration.com

SUTURING Part 1: The Principles and Techniques of Tying Knots
D. Oudit | M. Briggs

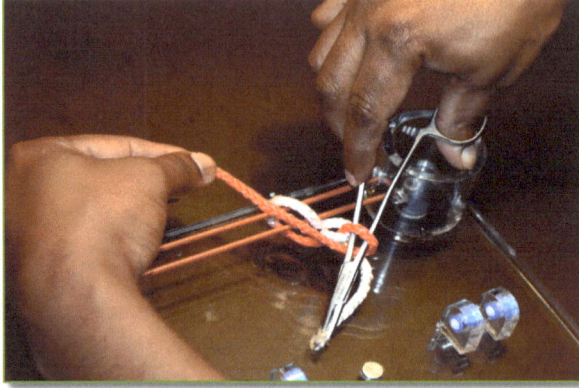

Step 6. The white end is then grasp by the tip of the haemostat.

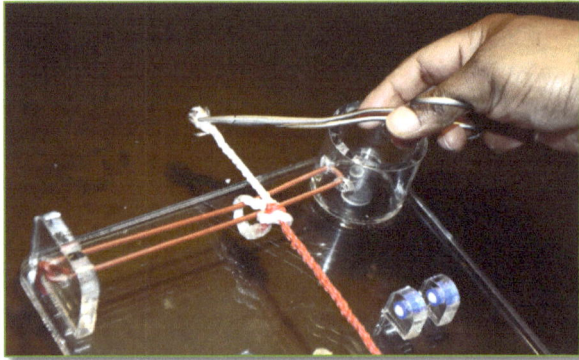

Step 7. Equal and horizontal tension is then applied to both ends with the red end being pulled towards the operator and the white end away from the operator. Note that both ends are now on the same sides as they were initially at the start.

This is the second throw completed.

This completes the **square knot**.

SurgicalIllustration.com

SUTURING Part 1: The Principles and Techniques of Tying Knots
D. Oudit | M. Briggs

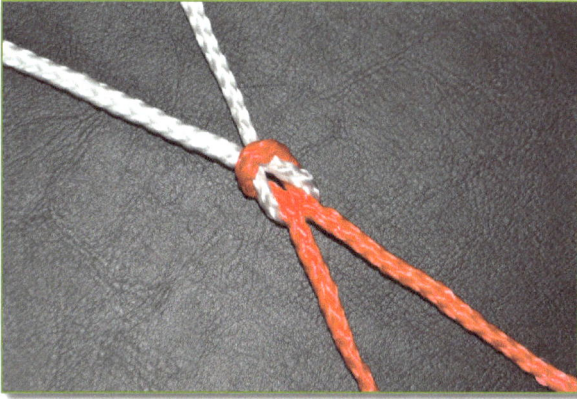

Figure 5.3. Note that the knot has both a symmetric and stable configuration.

CHAPTER 6

THE SURGEON'S KNOT

In this chapter the reader will study the properties of the surgeon's knot as well as the techniques of hand-tying and instrument tying this surgically popular knot.

Properties of the Surgeon's Knot:

- ✓ The surgeon's knot is a stable knot.
- ✓ It consists of at least two throws.
- ✓ It is useful as a tension knot.
- ✓ It is not as symmetrical as a square knot but can withstand more tension.
- ✓ It is slightly more bulky than the square knot.

The following figures demonstrate the technique of hand-tying a surgeon's knot - step by step.

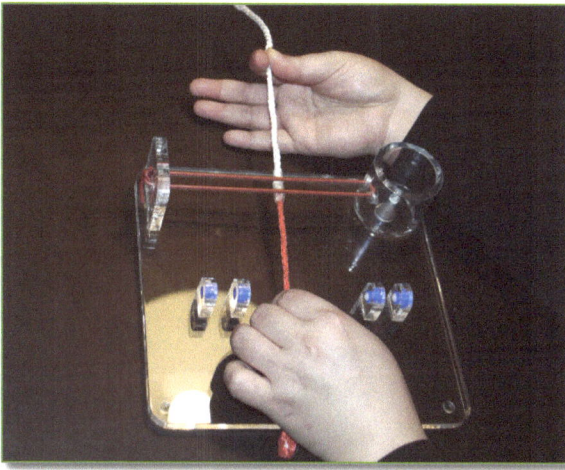

Step 1. The red end of the suture is held firmly between the thumb and index finger of the left hand in the pronated position. The white end of the suture is held firmly between the thumb and index finger of the right hand in the supinated position.

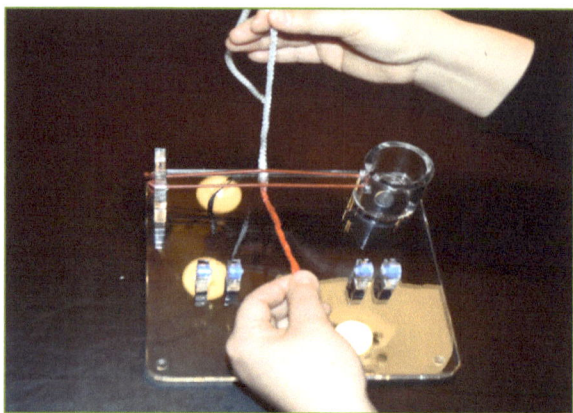

Step 2. Both hands are moved towards the middle of the field.

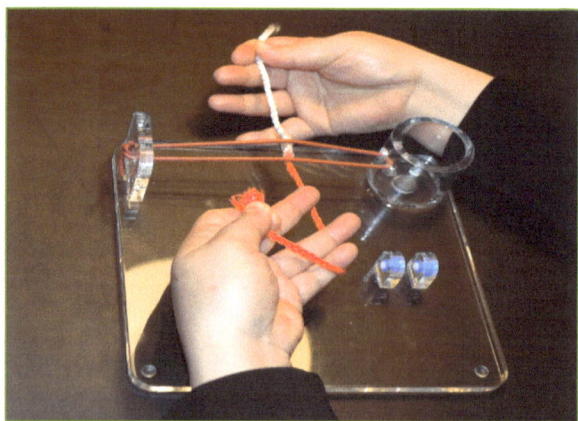

Step 3. The left hand is supinated with the red suture looping around the ulnar side of the little finger.

SUTURING Part 1: The Principles and Techniques of Tying Knots
D. Oudit | M. Briggs

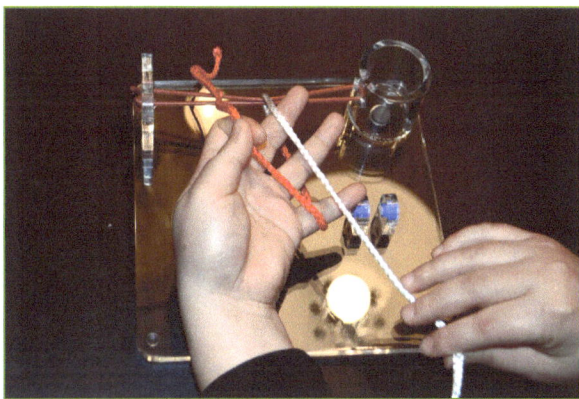

Step 4. The white end is brought to overlie the extended middle, ring and little fingers as shown.

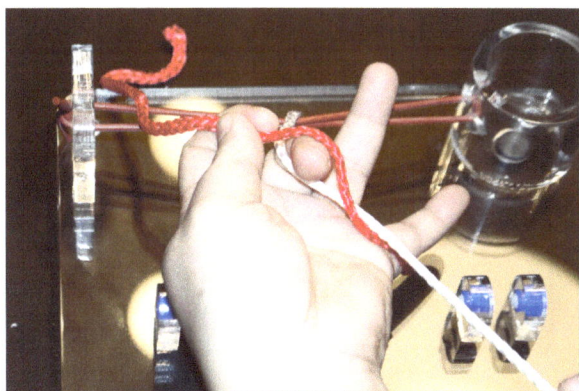

Step 5. The left middle finger is flexed over the white end and under the red end.

SUTURING Part 1: The Principles and Techniques of Tying Knots
D. Oudit | M. Briggs

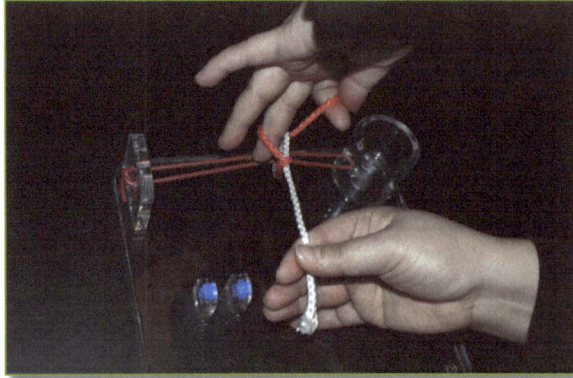

Step 6. The left hand is then pronated.

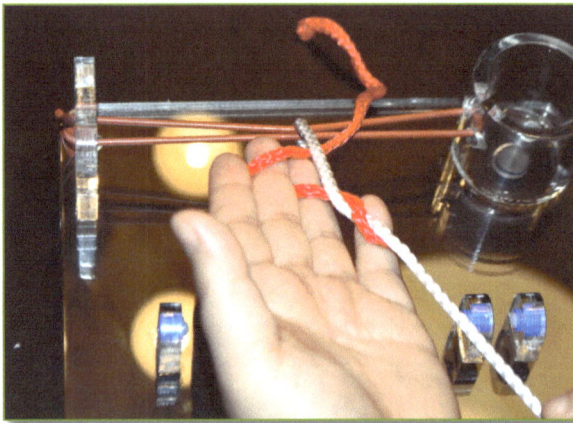

Step 7. The red end is then released by the left thumb and grasp between the left index and middle fingers. The left hand is then pronated and the left middle finger is passed under the white suture to grasp the end of the red suture. The red end is then brought under the white end.

SUTURING Part 1: The Principles and Techniques of Tying Knots
D. Oudit | M. Briggs

Another throw is performed.

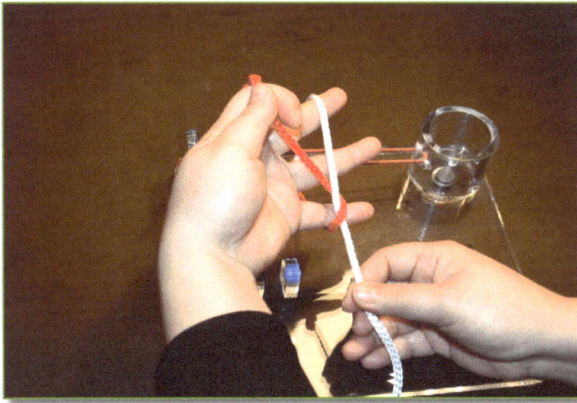

Step 8. The left extended left middle, ring and little fingers are inserted through the loop.

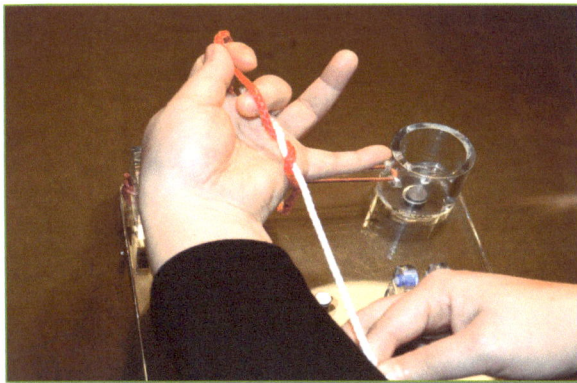

Step 9. The left middle finger is flexed over the white end.

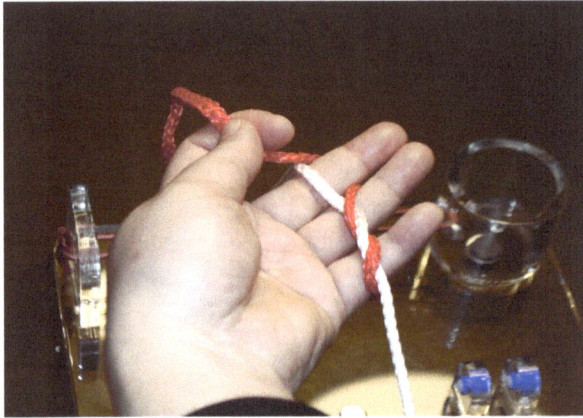

Step 10. The left middle finger is then extended over the red end.

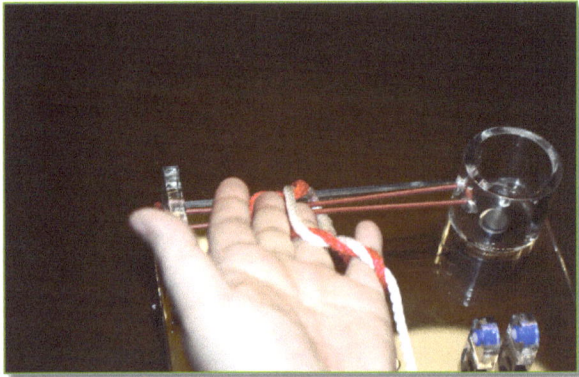

Step 11. The red end is then released by the left thumb and grasp between the left index and middle fingers and brought through under the white end.

SurgicalIllustration.com

SUTURING Part 1: The Principles and Techniques of Tying Knots
D. Oudit | M. Briggs

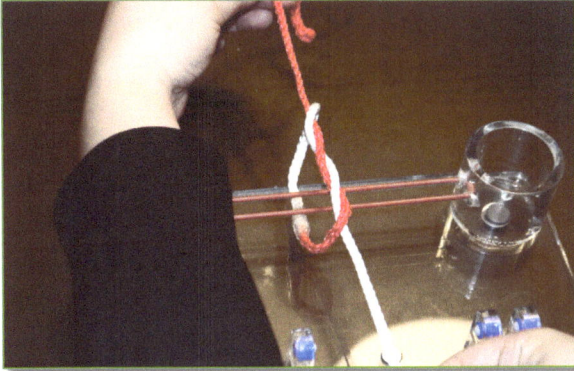

Step 12. Equal horizontal tension is then applied to both ends with the white end being pulled towards the operator and the red end away from the operator. Note that the ends are now on the opposite sides from where they initially started.

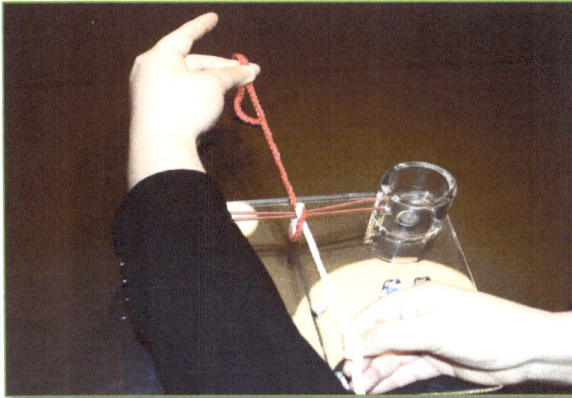

Step 13. The red end is now held between the left thumb and middle finger with the left hand in a pronated position. The white end is held between the right thumb and index finger with the right hand in a pronated position.

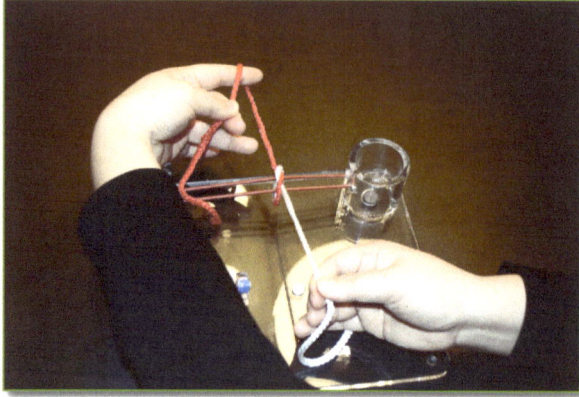

Step 14. The red and is then hooked the left index over the left index finger and brought towards to the middle of the field.

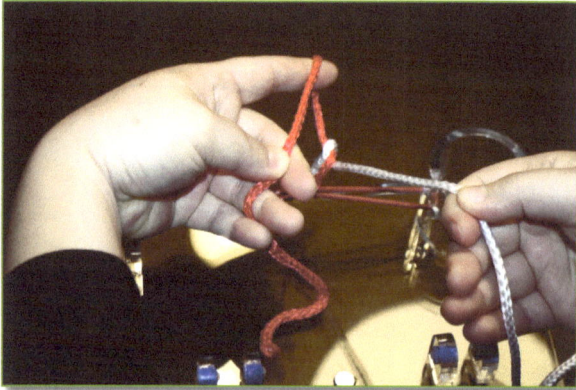

Step 15. The white end is also brought towards the middle of the field.

SurgicalIllustration.com

SUTURING Part 1: The Principles and Techniques of Tying Knots
D. Oudit | M. Briggs

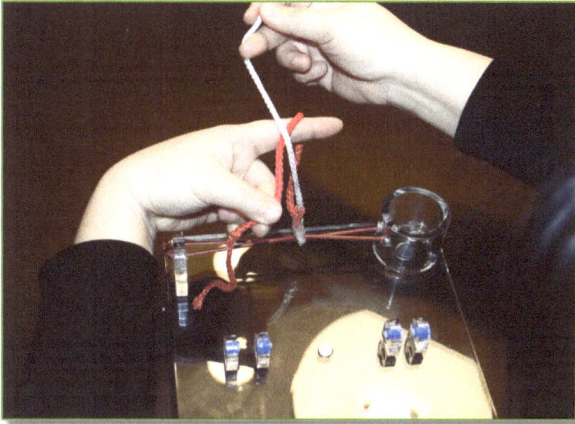

Step 16. The white end is brought to lie over the tip of the left index finger crossing the red end of the suture material.

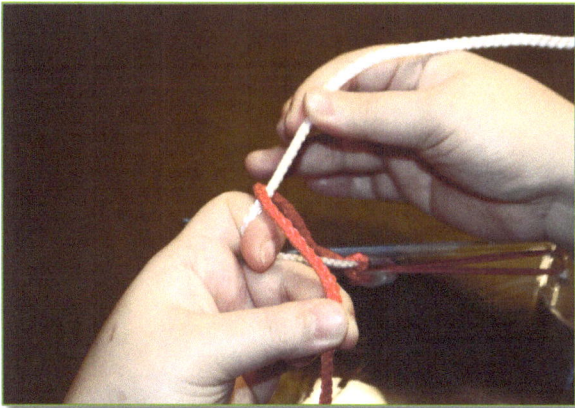

Step 17. The left index finger is then flexed over the white end pulling it inward and then extended over the red end to bring it under the white end.

Surgicalillustration.com

SUTURING Part 1: The Principles and Techniques of Tying Knots
D. Oudit | M. Briggs

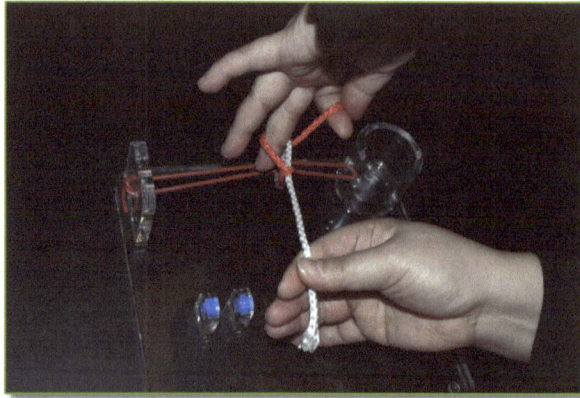

Step 18. The left hand is pronated.

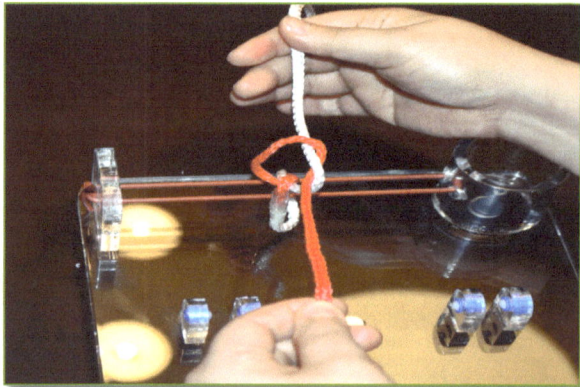

Step 19. The left hand is then pronated. The red end is released from the left thumb and middle fingers and the end pulled through under the white end. The red is then re-grasped between the left thumb and index and finger. Equal and horizontal tension is then applied with the red pulled towards the operator and the white away from the operator.

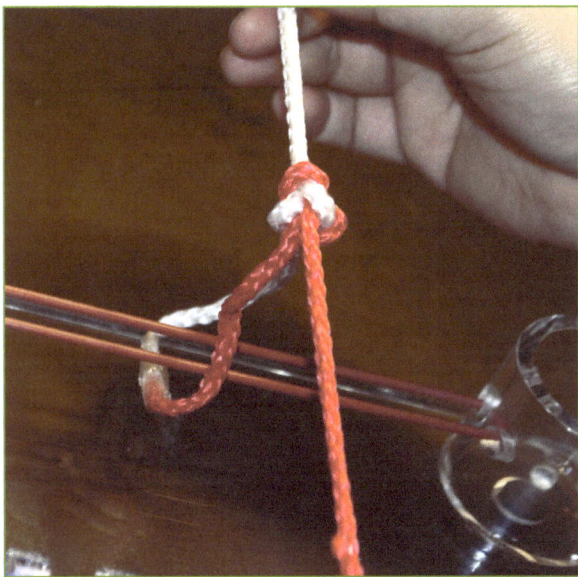

Figure 6.1: The configuration of the surgeon's knot. Note that it is a bit more bulky than the square knot.

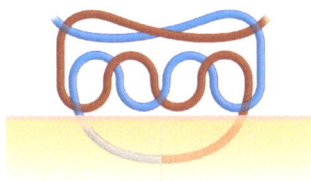

Figure 6.2: An illustration to highlight the configuration of the surgeon's knot.

INSTRUMENT-TYING THE SURGEON'S KNOT

SurgicalIllustration.com

SUTURING Part 1: The Principles and Techniques of Tying Knots
D. Oudit | M. Briggs

The following figures demonstrate the technique of tying a surgeon's knot using a haemostatic clamp or needle-holding forceps in a step-by-step fashion.

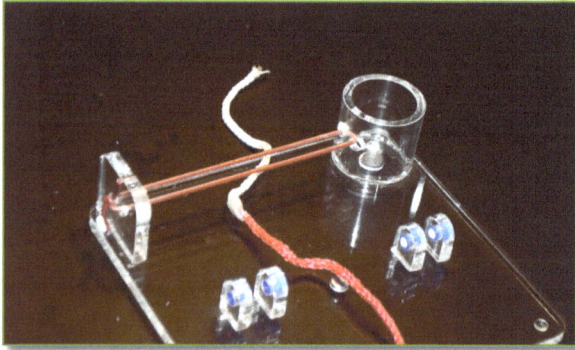

Step 1. The red end of the suture is held by one hand and a haemostatic clamp is held in the other hand. The white end of the suture is left free.

SurgicalIllustration.com

SUTURING Part 1: The Principles and Techniques of Tying Knots
D. Oudit | M. Briggs

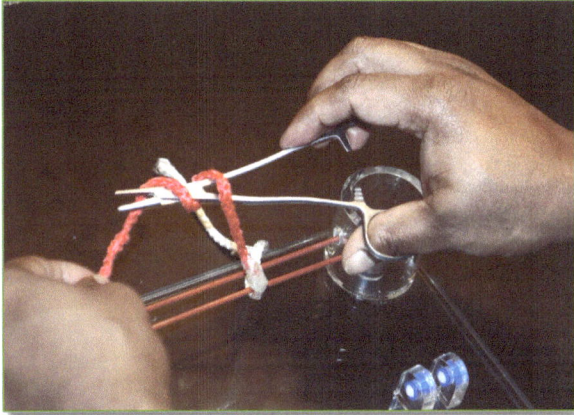

Step 2. The red end is looped around the tip of the haemostatic clamp twice in an anti-clockwise direction.

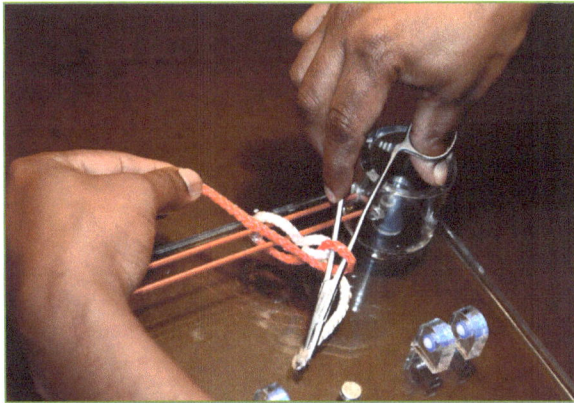

Step 3. The white end is then grasp by the tip of the haemostat.

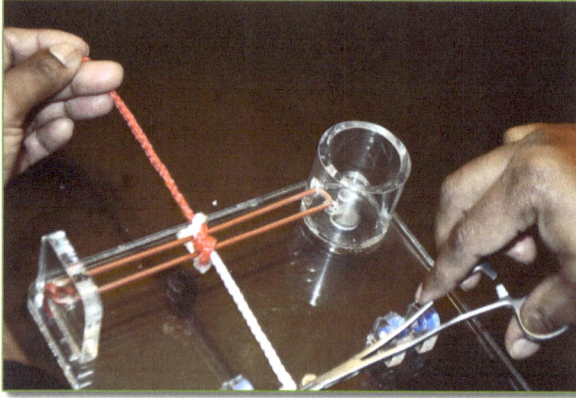

Step 4. Equal and horizontal tension is then applied to both ends with the white end being pulled towards the operator and the red end away from the operator. Note that the ends are now on opposite sides from they initially started.

This is the first throw completed. The second throw is illustrated below.

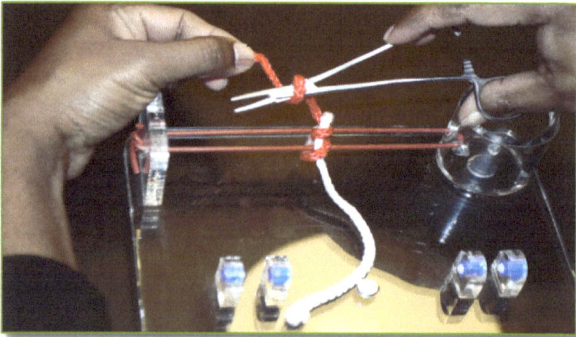

Step 5. The white end of the suture is then released from the tip of the haemostat. The red end is looped once around the tip of the haemostatic clamp in a clockwise direction.

SUTURING Part 1: The Principles and Techniques of Tying Knots
D. Oudit | M. Briggs

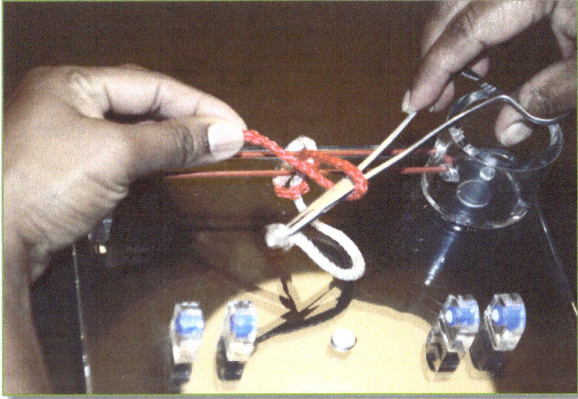

Figure 6. The white end is then grasp by the tip of the haemostat.

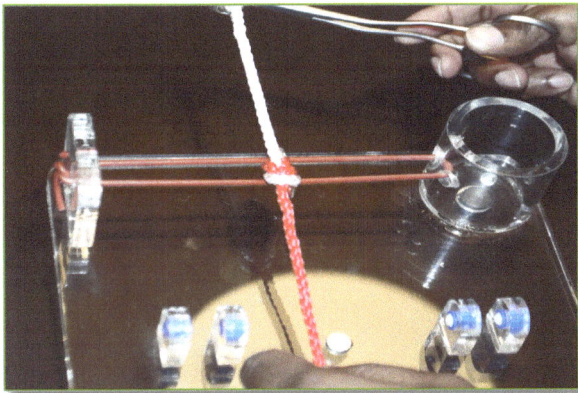

Figure 7. Equal and horizontal tension is then applied to both ends with the red end being pulled towards the operator and the white end away from the operator. Note that the ends are now back on the same sides from they initially started. This is the second throw completed.

CHAPTER 7

THE 'GRANNY KNOT'

INTRODUCTION

The 'Granny Knot' is a name give to inherently unstable knot. Its use is strongly discouraged in surgical practice. It is only mentioned in this chapter to warn readers of its use. The properties of a 'granny knot' are discussed below.

PROPERTIES OF THE 'GRANNY KNOT'

✓ The 'granny knot' is an inherently unstable knot.

✓ It is created by crossing of the suture strands incorrectly in the formation of a square knot resulting in an unstable configuration.

✓ It is asymmetric and more bulky than a square knot.

✓ It cannot withstand the tension.

SUTURING Part 1: The Principles and Techniques of Tying Knots

D. Oudit | M. Briggs

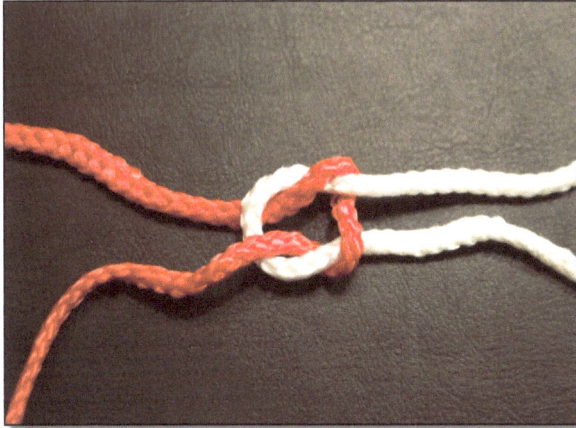

Figure 7.1: Configuration of the granny knot.

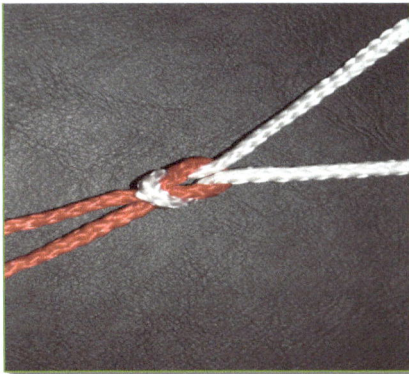

Figure 7.2: Configuration of the square knot for comparison.

SurgicalIllustration.com

SUTURING Part 1: The Principles and Techniques of Tying Knots
D. Oudit | M. Briggs

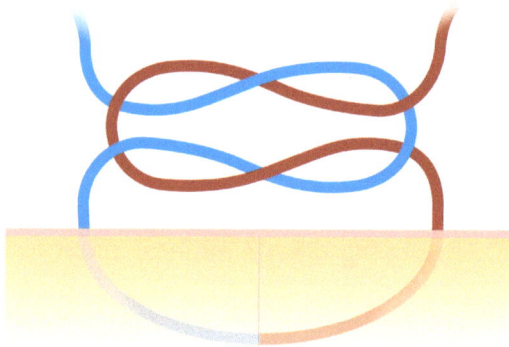

Figure 7.3: An illustration demonstrating the 'Granny Knot'.

CHAPTER 8

Tying a Knot in Deep Cavity

✓ This chapter outlines the technique of typing a stable knot in deep cavity as opposed to a wound on the skin surface.

✓ Tying a square knot in superficial tissues involve applying equal tension on the suture ends in a horizontal plane. In a deep cavity where space is limited this is more challenging.

✓ Care must taken while tying this knot such that too much tension on any one of the suture ends is not applied as this may result in avulsion of the tissues.

✓ It is critically important that the knot formed by this technique is stable.

SurgicalIllustration.com

SUTURING Part 1: The Principles and Techniques of Tying Knots
D. Oudit | M. Briggs

The following figures demonstrate the technique of hand-tying a square knot in a deep cavity in a step-by-step sequence. Please note that steps 1 to 10 are similar to those for the simple knot.

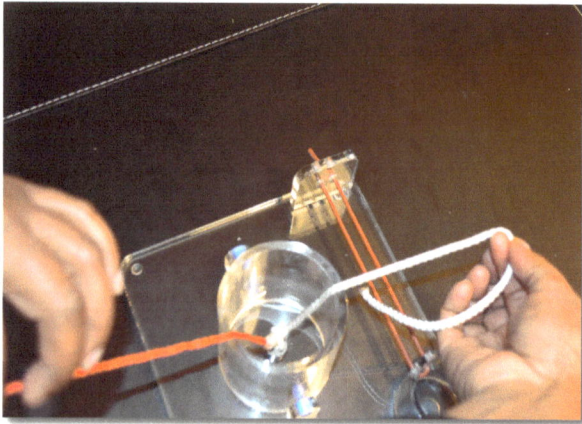

Step 1. Both ends of the strands are kept long. The red end of the suture is held firmly between the thumb and index finger of the left hand in the pronated position. The white end of the suture is held firmly between the thumb and index finger of the right hand in the supinated position.

SUTURING Part 1: The Principles and Techniques of Tying Knots
D. Oudit | M. Briggs

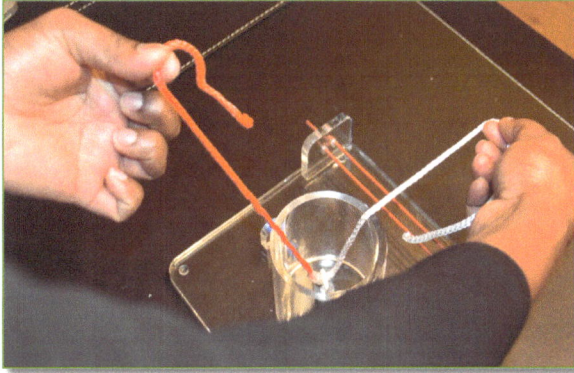

Step 2. Both hands are moved towards the middle of the field.

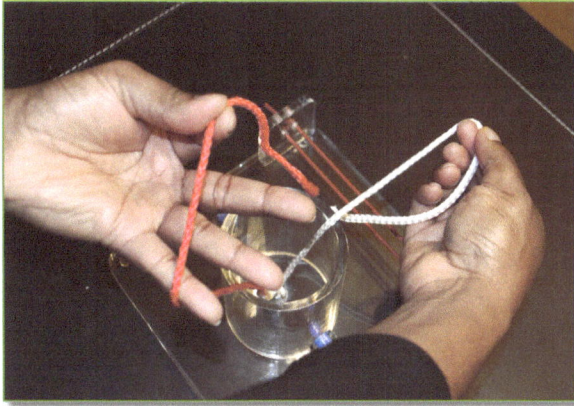

Step 3. The left hand is supinated with the ulnar 3 digits overlying the red suture hooking around the ulnar side of the little finger.

SurgicalIllustration.com

SUTURING Part 1: The Principles and Techniques of Tying Knots
D. Oudit | M. Briggs

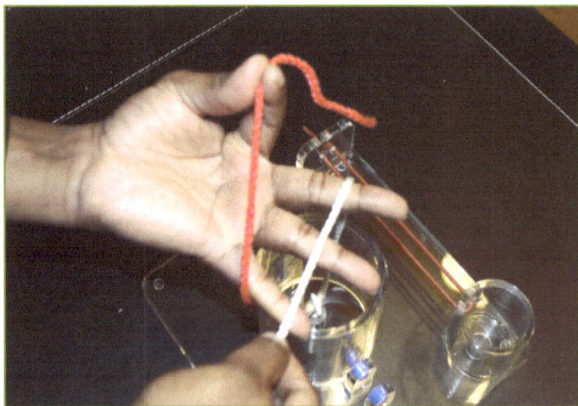

Step 4. The white end is brought to overlie the extended middle, ring and little fingers.

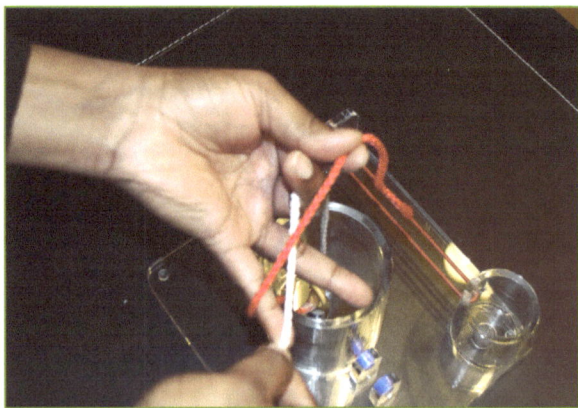

Step 5. The left middle finger is flexed over the white end.

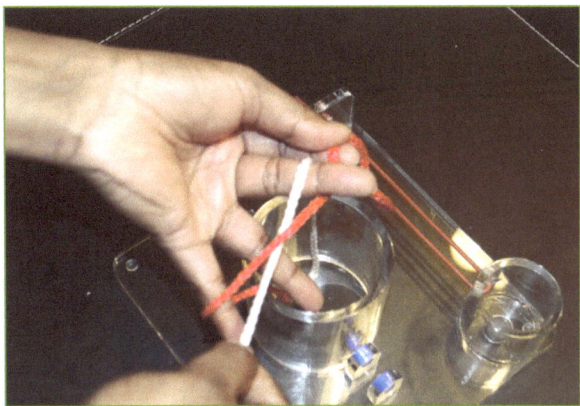

Step 6. Then the left middle finger is then extended over the red end.

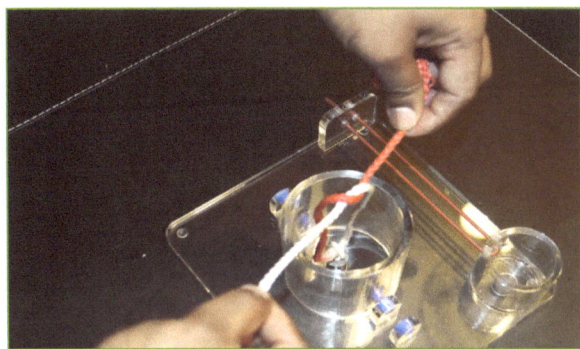

Step 7. The left hand is then pronated and the left thumb is passed under the white suture to grasp the end of the red suture. The red end is then brought under the white end. Equal and horizontal tension is then applied to both ends. Note that the ends are now on the opposite sides from where they initially started.

SurgicalIllustration.com

SUTURING Part 1: The Principles and Techniques of Tying Knots
D. Oudit | M. Briggs

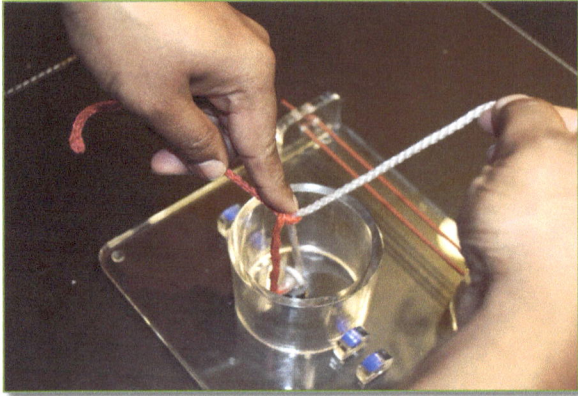

Step 8. The tip of the left index finger is placed on the red strand close to the knot and it is pushed down into the depth of the cavity while maintaining counter-tension on the white strand with the right hand. Final tension should be as horizontal as possible.

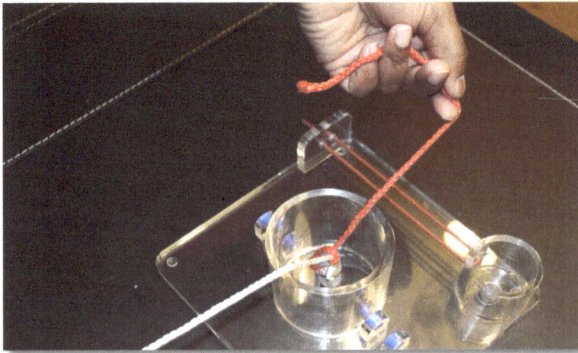

Step 9. Then the red strand is then grasped between the left thumb and index finger and the white strand by the right thumb and index finger.

SUTURING Part 1: The Principles and Techniques of Tying Knots
D. Oudit | M. Briggs

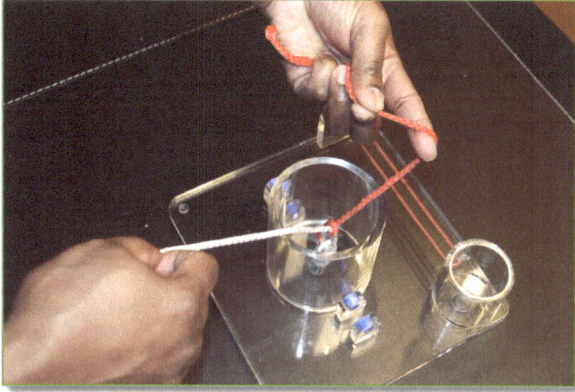

Step 10. The red and is then hooked the left index over the left index finger and brought towards to the middle of the field.

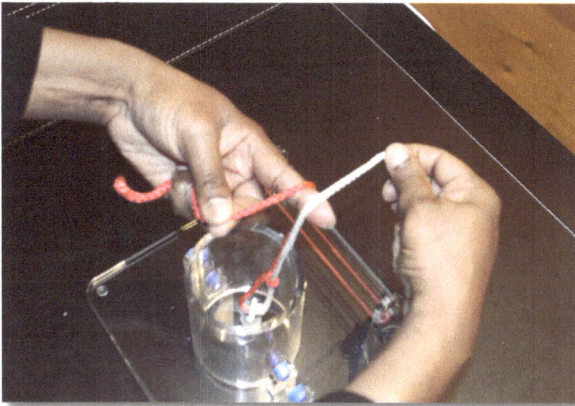

Step 11. The white end is brought to lie over the tip of the left index finger crossing the red end of the suture material.

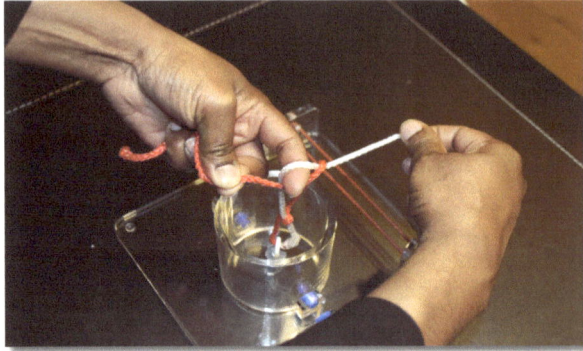

Step 12. The left index finger is then flexed over the white end pulling it inward and then extended over the red end to bring it under the white end.

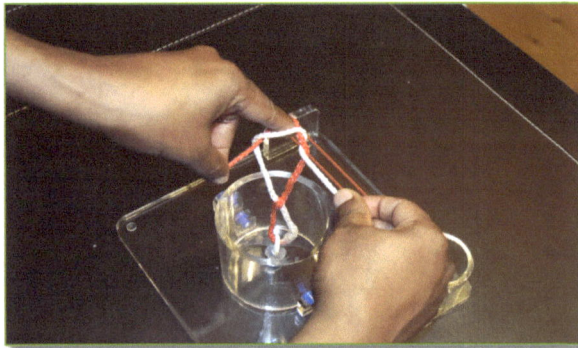

Step 13. The left hand is then pronated. The red end is released from the left thumb and middle fingers and the end pulled through under the white end. The red is then re-grasped between the left thumb and index and finger. Equal and horizontal tension is then applied with the red pulled towards the operator and the white away from the operator.

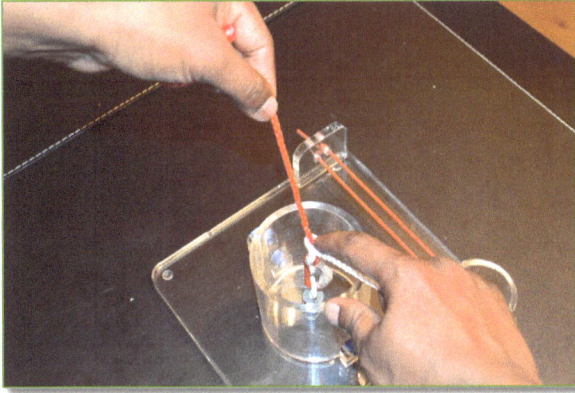

Step 14. This loop is advanced into the cavity by pushing on the white strand close to the loop while maintaining counter-tension on the red strand with the left hand.

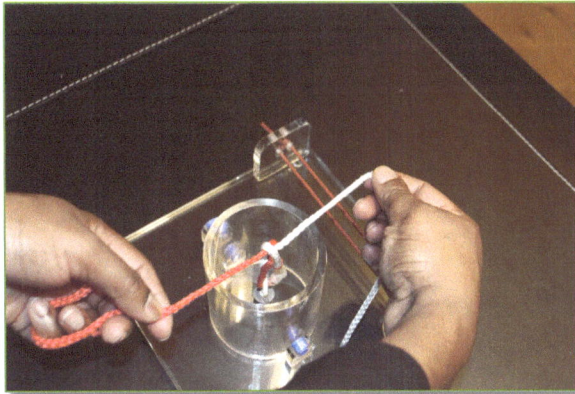

Step 15. Final tension should be as horizontal as possible with the left hand applying tension to the red end and the right hand to the right.

This completes a **square knot** in the deep cavity.

SurgicalIllustration.com

SUTURING Part 1: The Principles and Techniques of Tying Knots
D. Oudit | M. Briggs

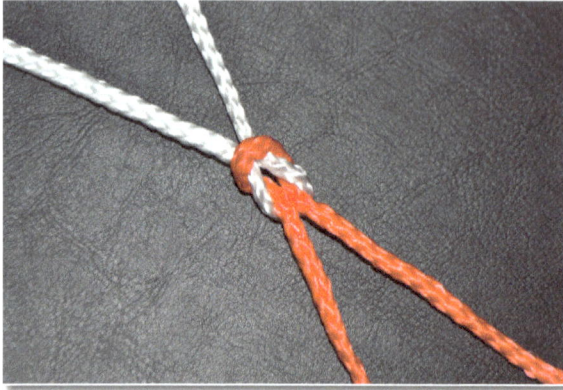

Figure 8.1: Note that the knot has both a symmetric and stable configuration.

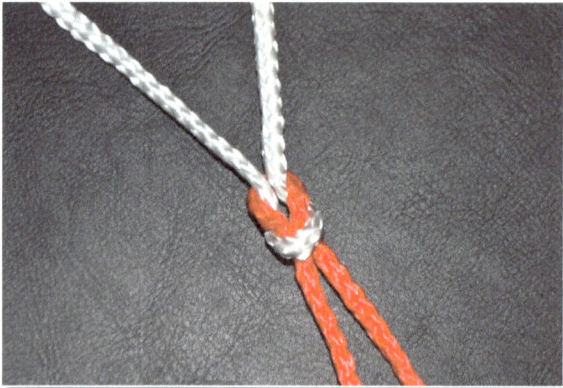

Figure 8.2: Note that the knot has both a symmetric and stable configuration.

CHAPTER 9

The 'Monkey on a Pole' Knot – An Unstable Knot

INTRODUCTION

- ✓ This knot is not recommended in surgical practice but is only outlined here to highlight the above. It is to be avoided.
- ✓ The 'Monkey on a Pole' knot involves tying an unstable knot in a deep cavity.
- ✓ The knot configuration is highly unstable and is easily demonstrated by pulling the vertical end on the suture material, which readily leads to unravelling the knot.
- ✓ This unstable knot is formed when the throws of a square knot are done repeated without alternating the suture end. As a result the throws are not 'locked'. This accounts for its instability.
- ✓ This results when only one strand is used to form the knots while vertical tension is applied to the other strand.
- ✓ The technique is described in the section below.

SurgicalIllustration.com

SUTURING Part 1: The Principles and Techniques of Tying Knots
D. Oudit | M. Briggs

The following figures demonstrate the technique of hand-tying this unstable knot step by step. Its use is discouraged from clinical practice.

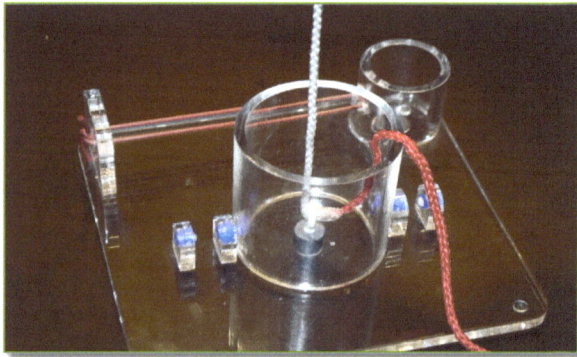

Step 1. Vertical tension applied to the white strand by the right hand.

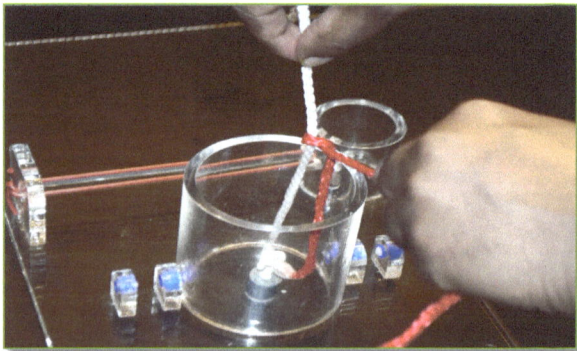

Step 2. The red strand is looped and advanced into the cavity with the left hand.

SUTURING Part 1: The Principles and Techniques of Tying Knots
D. Oudit | M. Briggs

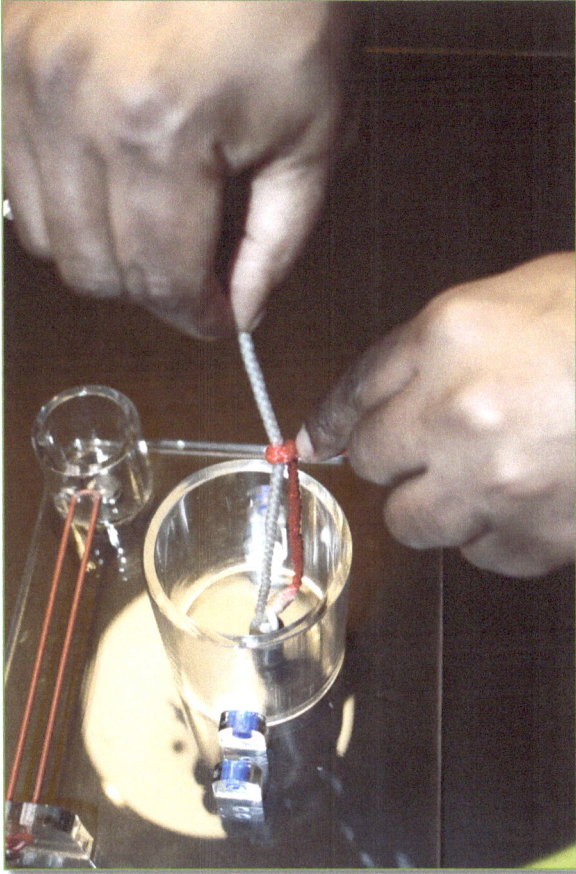

Step 3. The tip of the left index finger is then used to push the knot down the white suture into the cavity.

SurgicalIllustration.com

SUTURING Part 1: The Principles and Techniques of Tying Knots
D. Oudit | M. Briggs

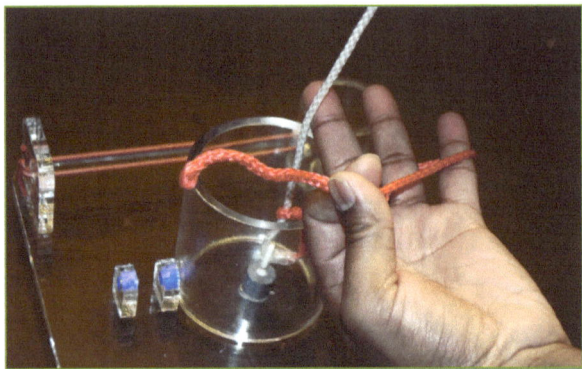

Step 4. The red strand is used again to create another throw in the same direction as the first with the left hand while still maintaining tension on the white strand with the right hand.

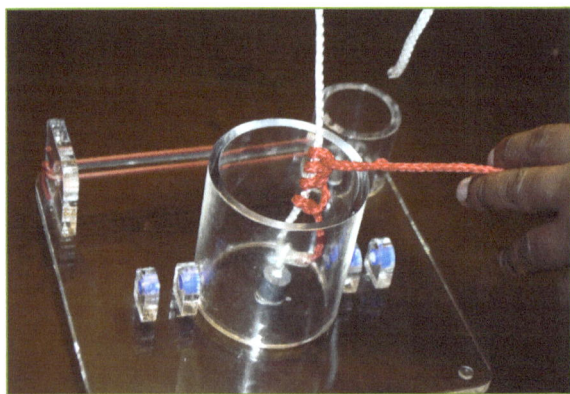

Step 5. Steps 1 - 4 are repeated several times.

[A]

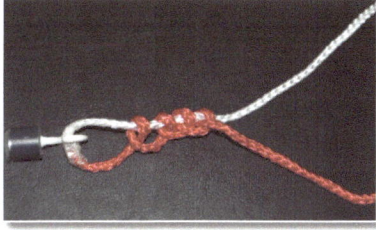

[B]

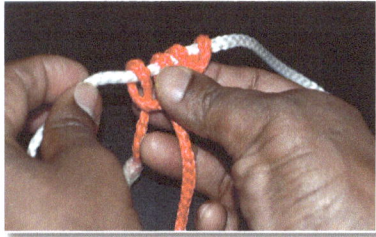

[C]

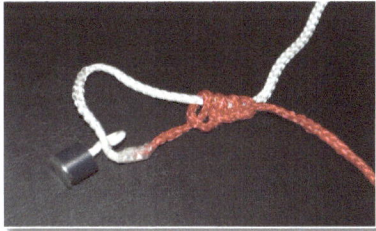

Figures 9.1 [A], [B] and [C]. This is a very unstable knot and can be easily unravelled. Its use is highly discouraged in surgical practice.

CHAPTER 10

Hand Tying a Square Knot Around a Haemostatic Clamp

INTRODUCTION

✓ This involves tying a square knot around the tip of the clamp that is attached to the free end of the divided vessel.

✓ The knot should consist of at least 2 throws.

✓ The knot formed should be stable.

HAND-TYING A SQUARE KNOT AROUND A HAEMOSTATIC CLAMP

The following figures demonstrate the technique of hand-tying a square around the tip of a haemostatic clamp in a step-by-step sequence.

SurgicalIllustration.com

SUTURING Part 1: The Principles and Techniques of Tying Knots
D. Oudit | M. Briggs

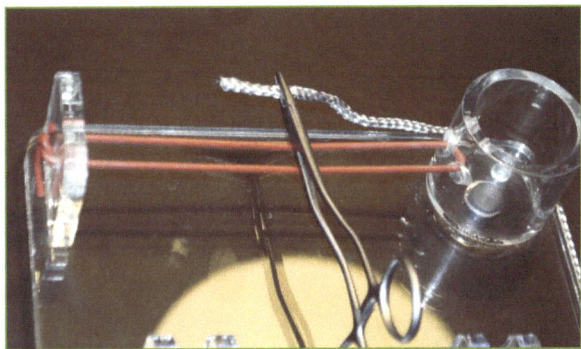

Step 1. The haemostatic clamp is placed gently and accurately grasping the vessel or tissue between its jaws. The tip of the clamp is allowed to project beyond the tissues. Care may be exercised to avoid injuring adjacent tissue in the process. The clamp is given to an assistant to control with its tip visible to the operator.

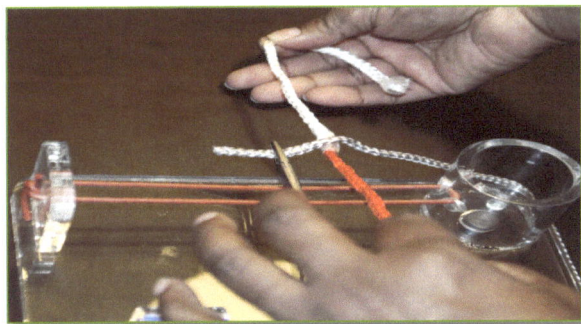

Step 2. A length of suture material is passed behind the clamp. The red end of the suture is held firmly between the thumb and index finger of the left hand in the pronated position. The white end of the suture is held firmly between the thumb and index finger of the right hand in the supinated position.

SurgicalIllustration.com

SUTURING Part 1: The Principles and Techniques of Tying Knots
D. Oudit | M. Briggs

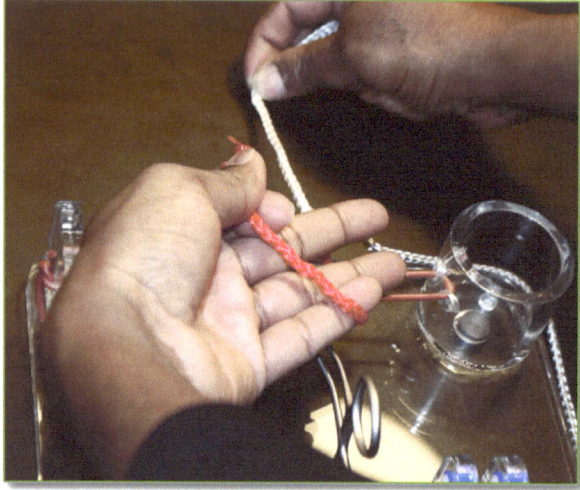

Step 3. The left hand is supinated over the red suture material.

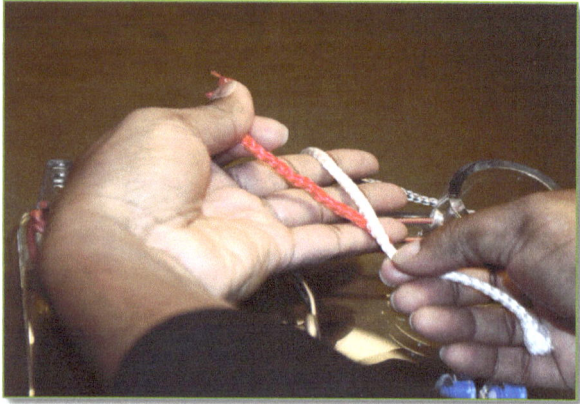

Step 4. The white end is brought to overlie the extended middle, ring and little fingers under the red end.

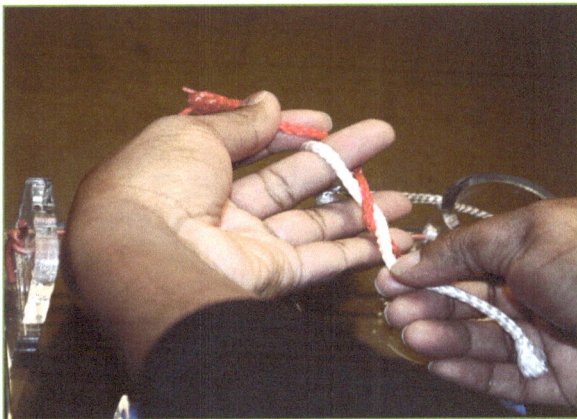

Step 5. The left middle finger is flexed over the white end and then extended over the red end.

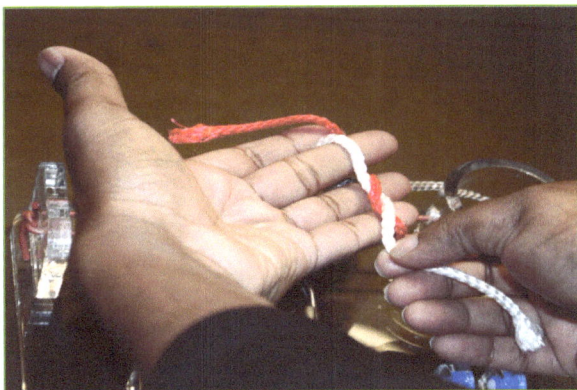

Step 6. The red end is then released by the left thumb and grasp between the left index and middle fingers.

SUTURING Part 1: The Principles and Techniques of Tying Knots
D. Oudit | M. Briggs

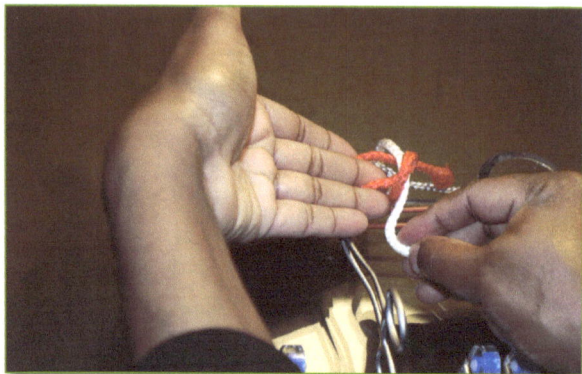

Step 7. The left hand is then pronated and the left middle finger is passed under the white suture to grasp the end of the red suture. The red end is then brought under the white end.

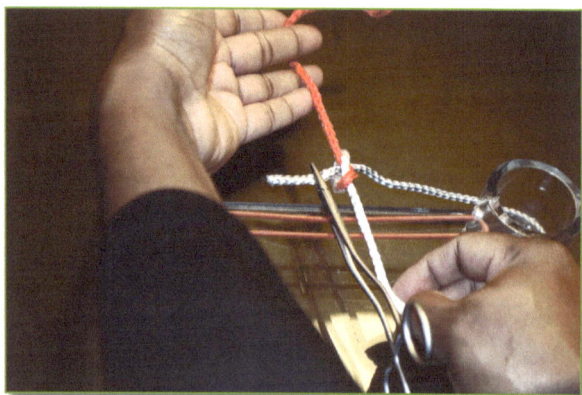

Step 8. Equal horizontal tension is then applied to both ends with the white end being pulled towards the operator and the red end away from the operator. Note that the ends are now on the opposite sides from where they initially started. Also, note that the knot is 'sitting' flat.

SurgicalIllustration.com

SUTURING Part 1: The Principles and Techniques of Tying Knots
D. Oudit | M. Briggs

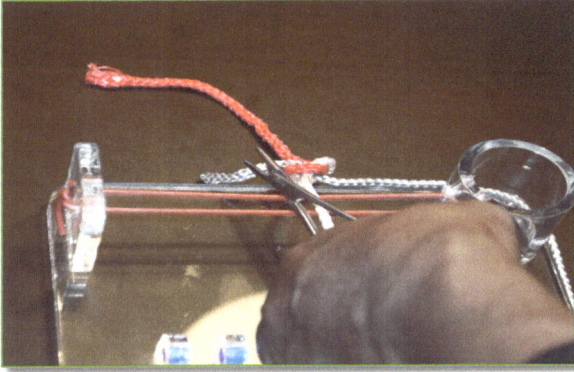

Step 9. The assistant is then instructed to remove the haemostatic clamp while tension is applied to the ends of the suture material.

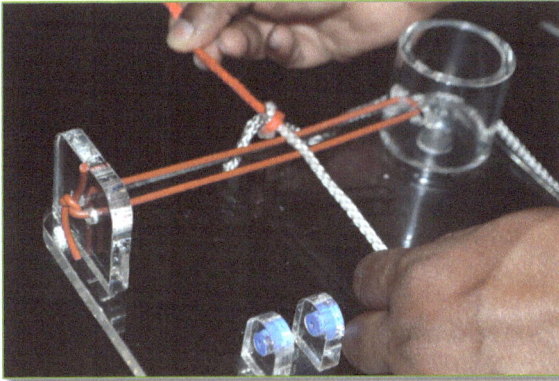

Step 10. The red end is now held between the left thumb and middle finger with the left hand in a pronated position. The white end is held between the right thumb and index finger with the right hand in a pronated position.

SurgicalIllustration.com

SUTURING Part 1: The Principles and Techniques of Tying Knots
D. Oudit | M. Briggs

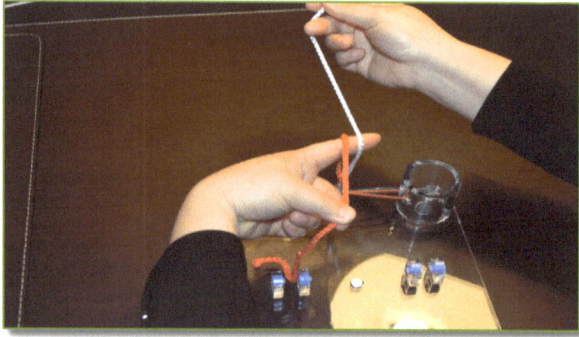

Step 11. The red and is then hooked the left index over the left index finger and brought towards to the middle of the field. The white end is brought towards the middle of the field crossing the red suture to lie over the tip of the left index finger.

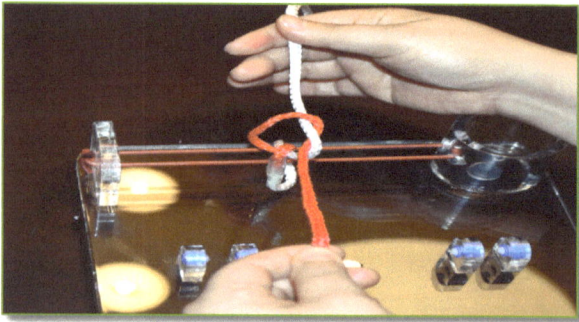

Step 12. The left index finger is then flexed over the white end pulling it inward and then extended over the red end to bring it under the white end. The red end is released from the left thumb and middle fingers and the end pulled through under the white end. The red is then re-grasped between the left thumb and index and finger. Equal and horizontal tension is then applied with the red pulled towards the operator and the white away from the operator.

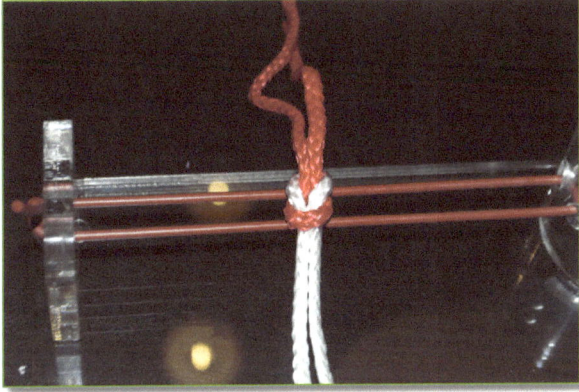

Figure 10.1. The completed knot is a square knot.

SurgicalIllustration.com

SUTURING Part 1: The Principles and Techniques of Tying Knots
D. Oudit | M. Briggs

CHAPTER 11

Instrument-Tying a Knot Around a Haemostatic Clamp

✓ This involves tying a square knot around the tip of the clamp that is attached to the free end of the divided vessel using a needle-holder using a needle-holding forceps and a haemostatic clamp.

✓ The knot formed should be a square knot which stable.

✓ This has the advantage of saving on suture material and is recommended where possible.

✓ The technique is described in the section below.

The following figures demonstrate the technique of tying a square knot around the tip of a haemostatic clamp using a haemostatic clamp or needle-holding forceps in a step-by-step fashion.

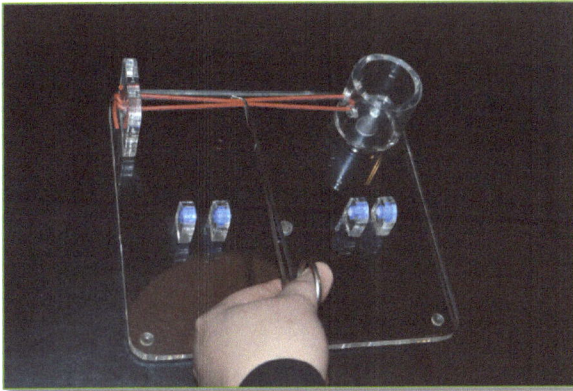

Step 1. The haemostatic clamp is placed gently but accurately grasping the vessel or tissue between its jaws. The tip of the clamp is allowed to project beyond the tissues. The clamp is given to an assistant to control with the tip of the clamp visible to the operator.

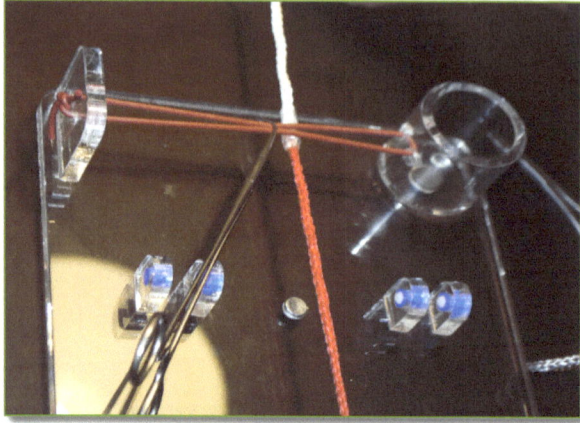

Step 2. A length of suture material is passed behind the clamp.

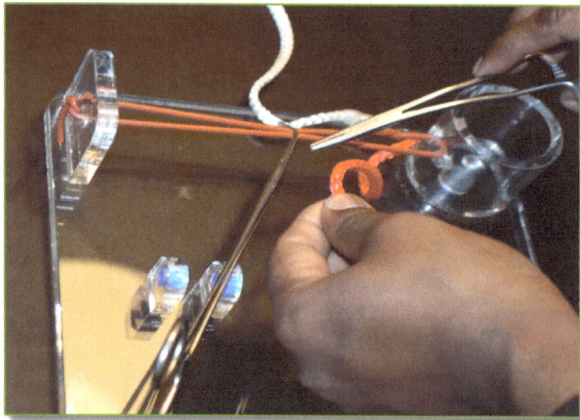

Step 3. The red end of the suture is held by one hand and a haemostatic clamp is held in the other hand. The white end of the suture is left free.

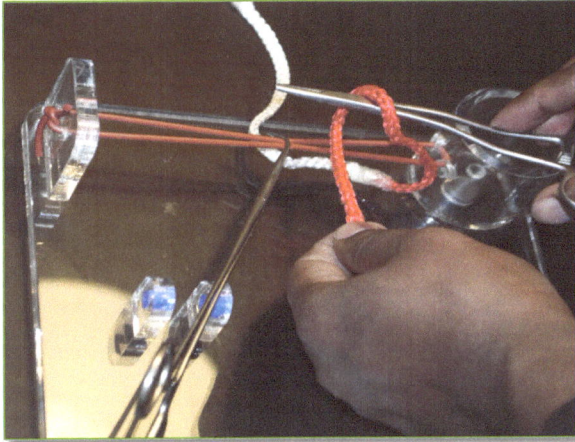

Step 4. The red end is looped around the tip of the haemostatic clamp.

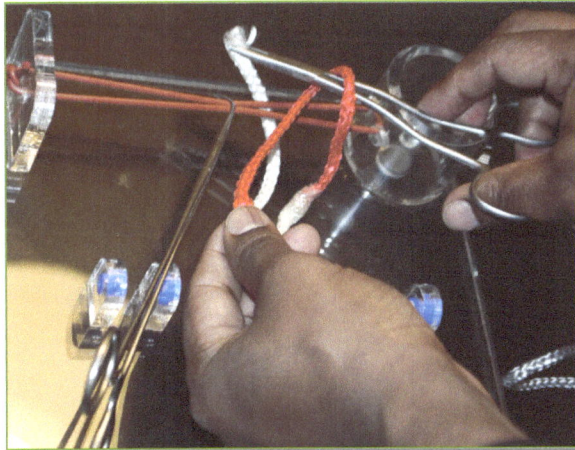

Step 5. The white end is then grasp by the tip of the haemostat.

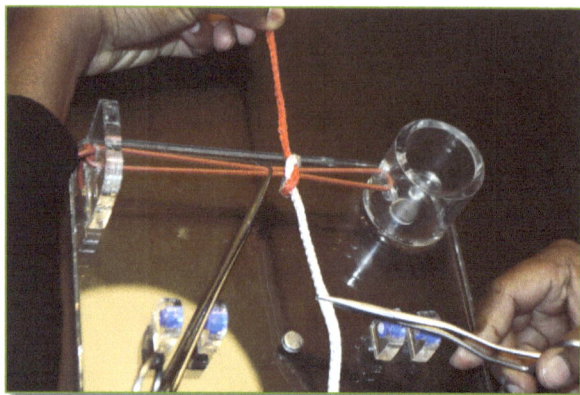

Step 6. Equal and horizontal tension is then applied to both ends with the white end being pulled towards the operator and the red end away from the operator. Note that the ends are now on opposite sides from they initially started.

This is the first throw completed.

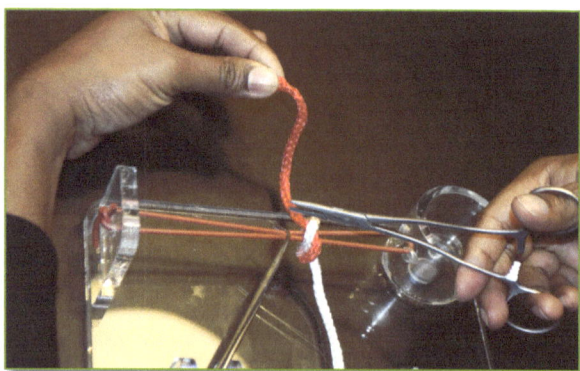

Step 7. The white end of the suture is then released from the tip of the haemostat.

SUTURING Part 1: The Principles and Techniques of Tying Knots
D. Oudit | M. Briggs

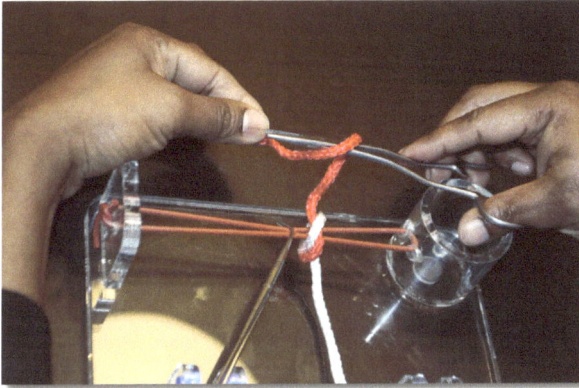

Step 8. The red end is looped around the tip of the haemostatic clamp in a clockwise direction.

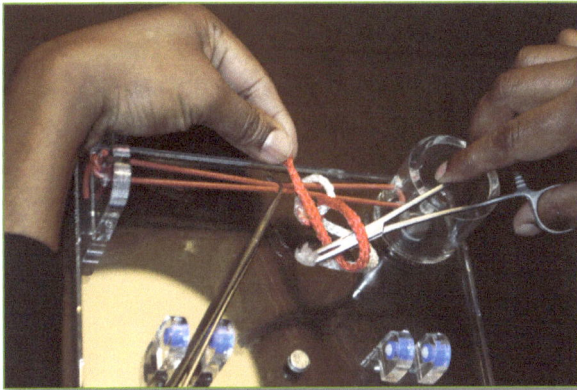

Step 9. The white end is then grasp by the tip of the haemostat.

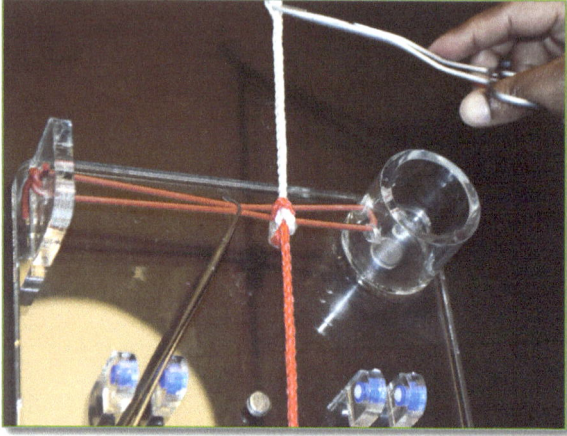

Step 10. Equal and horizontal tension is then applied to both ends with the red end being pulled towards the operator and the white end away from the operator. Note that the ends are now back on the same sides from they initially started.

Index

SurgicalIllustration.com

SUTURING Part 1: The Principles and Techniques of Tying Knots
D. Oudit | M. Briggs